Judith Wills is one of Britain's best-known diet and fitness writers. She was editor of *Slimmer* magazine for ten years and went on to run a weekly slimming column in the Daily Express. Author of the bestselling *A Flat Stomach in 15 Days* and *High Speed Slimming*, Judith also broadcasts regularly on television and radio.

SIZE
12
in
21
Days

Judith Wills

ARROW

Note: The size 12 referred to in this book is the British size 12. The equivalent American and European sizes are 10 and 40 respectively.

To Mother
with love and thanks

Published in 1993 by Vermilion Arrow
an imprint of Ebury Press
Random House UK Ltd
20 Vauxhall Bridge Road
London SW1V 2SA

1 3 5 7 9 10 8 6 4 2

A catalogue record for this book is available from the British Library

Printed and bound in Great Britain by Cox & Wyman Ltd., Reading, Berkshire

ISBN 0 09 923421 1

CONTENTS

ACKNOWLEDGEMENTS

Many thanks for all your valuable input and hard work to: Jan Bowmer and all the editorial team, to Dennis Barker and the Design team and to Niccy Cowen and Gina Rozner.

Heartfelt thanks to Tony for your encouragement and support, and for everything you did to ensure Size 12 was finished on time. And thanks also for so much patience in photographing the exercises!

Thank you to Bodyline Dancewear, 67a Elm Grove, Southsea, Hants (tel: 0705 824921) for supplying me with a large selection of exercise clothes.

And thanks also to Jane Turnbull; Lamberts of Hereford; Sheena at Keith and Peter; Chris, William and Louise Court.

INTRODUCTION

There's no doubt about it, thin is no longer in. For the woman of the '90s, her shape to be is ... well ... shapely.

And so *Size 12 in 21 Days* is the first diet book for women who don't want to be thin. It's written for women like you and me – women who want to look good but aren't afraid to be female. We want a bust, a waist, hips and a bottom. We want the shape that fits into – and looks great in – a size-12 dress.

Today's clothes actually look better on a fuller figure – those stretchy leggings need a bottom, the low-cut tops need a bust, and all those lycra dresses need curves, not bones. That's why all the most in-demand catwalk models are a size 12, too. Ten years ago, the standard for models was an 8, at most a 10. Twiggy was 32-22-32 ins (80-55-80 cm). Today she'd need to have a 36-inch (91 cm) bust and 36-inch (91 cm) hips to stand a chance!

Thank goodness that finally we've come to realize that being thin and shapeless is neither ideal nor even possible for most of us. Achieving size 12 is, I can assure you, much easier, much more feasible and much, much more satisfying than aiming for a specific, unrealistic low-target weight. How many of us have painfully pruned away every last ounce down to a pre-determined 'target', only to discover that we still felt dissatisfied with the way we looked – either because the weight had gone from the wrong places, or else we were left thin but, somehow, still 'baggy'.

And, although I'm sure you'll feel delighted when you

can walk into your local boutique and head for the size-12 rails, rather than being made to feel like an elephant when you head towards the dark size-16 corner, getting into a 12 isn't just a matter of vanity. That's because your dress size is usually a better indication of your fitness and health than your weight is. A slim waist and taut stomach indicate a fit, well-toned, healthy body, whatever you weigh. The distribution of your weight – your statistics – is the real key to how you look and feel. And that is what this book is all about – shape, tone, size and proportion. You will lose weight, certainly, if you're slimming down whole dress sizes, but you may not need to lose as much weight as you think.

Let me give you a personal example. For two years or so after the birth of one of my children, I took a size 16 in all clothes that had a waistband – the result of having a 30-inch (75 cm) or so waist. Yet, at 5 ft 7 ins (1.7 m), I weighed only 9 stone 12 lbs (64 kg), well within my limit on those 'weight for height' charts.

I used to dream of getting down to 8½ stone (55 kg), like the models of my own height I was always reading about. But gradually I came to realize that I wasn't made or meant to be 8½ stone (55 kg). Instead, I worked on my shape while I ate a diet of the right kinds of foods. In the end I'd lost just 10 lbs (4.6 kg) in all before I could fit easily into a 12 – a size I don't find it difficult to maintain. In other words, what I did was change my size and shape – from 37-30-37 ins (92-75-92 cm) down to 36-26-36 ins (90-65-90 cm) while losing only 5 lbs (2.3 kg) per dress size! I know many women who have lost 1½ or 2 stones (9.5 or 13 kg) and still didn't get down two dress sizes!

Size 12 is not an impossible goal – for most of us it is a real possibility. Size 12 is within the grasp of every out-of-shape woman, whether you're a 14, 16, or more.

Remember: with the Size 12 in 21 Days system, you may not need to lose as much weight as you think. Yes, you'll lose some weight, so I'm not going to ask you to throw out your bathroom scales. But the system works, and works quickly, because it doesn't just depend on weight loss alone.

The diet is a tasty, no-hunger plan that works to shed fat quickly for people who most need it because of its special, high-carbohydrate, snacking system. But what you will also learn is how to contour your body into that size-12 shape by a simple, 20-minute exercise system that concentrates on the parts that affect your dress size the most – bust, waist, stomach, hips and bottom. And, because of a back-up system of mini-programmes, you can also give extra attention to your own trouble spots – a boon for so many of us who find they have a size-12 bust and waist but size-14 hips, or a size-12 bust and hips but size-16 waist!

Even better, you literally will be melting body fat from stomach, hips, bottom and thighs with the fat-burning routine – an easy yet effective, graded walking programme.

In other words, the system works quickly by allowing you to lose weight, by burning fat from where it needs to go, and by re-shaping and tightening your contours. These tactics can produce rapid body measurement improvements.

And, lastly, you'll discover how to look inches slimmer almost instantly when you learn the art of body awareness and correct body alignment.

By the way, if you happen to be very petite – say, under 5 ft 3 ins (1.6 m) – the system will work just as well to reduce you from a 12 down to a 10. Or, if you're very tall, say, 5 ft 8 ins (1.73 m) or over, it will work to reduce you from a 16 or an 18 down to a 14, which may well be your perfect size. Just follow the same diet and activity programme, but read your special notes on pages 22–23, first.

You can, of course, use the *Size 12 in 21 Days* programme, whatever dress size you currently take – 18, 20, or more – but obviously the more dress sizes you need to lose, the more times you will need to repeat the programme. It is, however, perfectly safe to follow for as long as you need to.

Once you've achieved your target size, you'll find it easy to maintain your new shape with the help of the comprehensive maintenance programme. It explains all you need to know to keep your size-12 figure for ever.

Before you start, let me assure you that if you follow the programme with enthusiasm you will see fantastic results. This book is not the programme for you if you're feeling half-hearted. It needs commitment and determination because it is a programme that asks you to do something for your body every day. But I believe that a concentrated effort is often easier to achieve than a lazier, but often never-ending, diet regime.

Size 12 in 21 Days is specially designed to work for you. It is a celebration of the curvier woman. So if you want the shape of today, start straight away. You'll be glad you did.

Chapter 1
THE 21-DAY PROGRAMME

—— YOUR DAILY SCHEDULE ——

In just 21 days from now, you can be up to two dress sizes smaller, with a body shape of which you can at last be really proud.

The 21-day schedule in this chapter outlines your complete diet programme. The schedule also sets out a carefully graded activity programme for you to follow, which is designed to change your shape speedily but safely.

Before you begin the schedule it is important that you read the diet and activity notes and instructions that follow below.

The Diet

The 21-day diet is not in any way a crash diet, nor a fad diet. It is a healthy, low-fat diet and it is within government healthy eating guidelines on every nutritional aspect. The diet is also 'user-friendly', relying in the main on simple produce, with the accent on meals that are quick to prepare yet high on taste.

Expected weight loss

The exact amount of weight you will lose on this programme depends upon several factors, including your personal metabolism, your body composition (the percentage of actual fat your body contains) and your starting weight. But, generally, the more fat you need to lose, the more pounds you will shed on the 21-day programme.

If, on the other hand, your measurements are due more to poor body tone or posture faults, the scales may register a smaller loss, but the activity programme will produce the measurement reduction you are looking forward to.

To shed two dress sizes – say, from a 16 to a 12 – most women need to lose up to a stone (6.4 kg), but don't keep hopping on to the scales while you're on the programme. Weight loss is not the same as 'size loss', which is why I want you to weigh yourself only on the days specified in the programme. I also want you to measure yourself regularly, too. This is one diet and exercise programme where the tape measure is more important than the scales!

The no-hunger way to diet

One benefit of my 21-day diet that I should mention right here is that you needn't fear the dreaded hunger pangs. Although the programme will produce quick weight loss if it's needed – particularly quick fat loss – it won't allow you to become hungry, because it is high in carbohydrates that keep you feeling full for longer. Also, snacks are allowed during the day so you never have to go too long without eating.

Another benefit of a high-carbohydrate diet is that carbohydrates convert themselves to energy in your body (i.e., burn themselves off) much more readily than do the calories in fat. And they actually speed up your metabolic rate, helping you to lose weight more quickly than on most other diets – without having to take those calories too low.

12

Bonus benefits

There are several more benefits to the special 21-day diet that you will discover.

- You'll feel better! If you have been eating a diet low in nutritious goodies, such as vitamins, minerals, and fresh fruits and vegetables, you may well have been feeling below par for some time – lacking in energy, sluggish, maybe a little depressed. This diet will help you to have more vitality and energy.

- Your skin, hair, gums, eyes and nails will improve. Eating well doesn't just mean losing weight, your whole body, from top to toe, can change for the better! Within the 21 days you'll probably see whiter eyes, healthier gums and better, clearer skin. Longer term, hair may become glossier, nails grow stronger, and so on.

- Many minor, and not-so-minor, ailments will improve or clear up altogether because of a combination of better diet and exercise. PMT, fluid retention, low blood sugar, digestive problems, constipation and other niggling problems can be helped through a good, healthy diet.

- On the 21-day diet you will learn good eating habits and overcome problems such as bingeing. A combination of the carbohydrate factor and the addition of regular snacks will help you to control any urge to binge. And that brings me on to the last great benefit of the diet.

- You'll have no problem making the transition from a reduced-calorie diet to a maintenance diet. The principles of the Size-12 diet are principles you will want to follow for the rest of your life. For more on weight maintenance, turn to Chapter 6.

——THE 21 DAYS IN DETAIL——

Let's go through each of the 21 days and see just how the diet works to get the fat moving off you so quickly.

The tough start

On Days 1 and 2 only, you will be following a strict, but delicious, diet. Both days contain a maximum of 600 calories a day.

I've chosen this 'tough start' for three reasons; one is psychological. At the start of any diet programme, your enthusiasm and determination is always very high. By starting off 'tough' we cash in on that feeling. You'll easily be able to sail through the two tough days, knowing there is much more food to come on Day 3!

Another reason is physical: these two days will produce a very significant weight loss, part of which will be tissue fluid and glycogen (the body's store of glucose-type instant energy). This loss will be most noticeable around your stomach and waist; therefore, by the end of Day 2, you should already be able to see a reduction in your measurements.

And the third reason is conditional. You will find, after two days of eating lovely, fresh, low-salt, low-fat foods, that you have literally given your taste buds a crash course in enjoying good, healthy foods rather than fatty, salty, over-sweet foods.

Days 3–7 The rest of the first week will be a doddle for you, calorie-wise. After the tough start, the schedule keeps you from straying by taking you straight up to its eating peak of 1100 or so calories a day. These extra calories are all good, healthy calories, consisting mainly of carbohydrate-rich foods, so you will still be educating your taste buds in the right way.

At the end of the first week you can weigh yourself; you'll find a loss of up to 6 lbs (2.7 kg) on average. (If you have stones to lose, the loss could be more.) The best news of all is that you may already be able to get into one dress size smaller!

Days 8–14 Now, gradually, we begin to reduce the calories again to keep the weight moving off. This week you will be on a steady 950 calories per day – all easy-to-prepare, delicious meals that will help you to lose up to 5 lbs (2.3 kg) this week as you see your vital statistics head towards their target.

Days 15–21 We're going down further to finish the diet on a week at 800 calories a day. However, it will seem as if you are eating much more than that and I promise you that you still won't feel hungry. You will find this last week of the diet easy – and you'll register a weight loss of around 3 lbs (1.4 kg), giving you a total loss of up to 14 lbs (6.4 kg) for the three-week period.

Diet instructions

It's important to follow these instructions, which should be applied throughout all the days of the 21-day diet.

- Try to space your meals evenly throughout the day.
- Never skip a meal.
- Eat everything you are allowed. If you don't eat something you are allowed – say, a piece of fruit at mid-morning – then be sure to eat it later in the day.
- When a recipe is given for a meal, there is always a simpler (sometimes quicker) plain meal option. Choose whichever you prefer.

• All recipes serve two but quantities can usually be halved for one – or doubled for four. Often, recipes can be frozen; if you are on your own it's worth cooking a two-portion serving and freezing half.

• The diet is suitable for most people, whether you live alone or have a family. Non-dieting members of the family can eat the same food but they can have bigger portions, or additions; e.g., more bread or potatoes.

• Vegetarians can follow the diet. There are many suitable vegetarian meals within the diet, and when there is a meal that includes meat, poultry or fish without a vegetarian alternative given, it is perfectly fine to substitute a low-fat vegetarian option; e.g., tofu, soya mince, vegeburger, beans or a low-fat cheese.

• The food charts at the back of this book will help you work out portion sizes. Always include all the accompaniments listed with the meal.

• Some people say dieting is expensive. While some of the items within this diet may seem more expensive than what you usually eat, the total cost of the diet works out at no more – and usually less – than the average person spends on food. This is because I have frequently used lower-cost items such as pulses, potatoes and grains, and also because you will be cutting out many of the foods you were eating before – saving a fortune on items such as biscuits, cakes and so forth!

• Most people have one or two food items on which they are not keen, or perhaps to which they are allergic. If a food item which you truly can't eat appears in the diet, then you can do one of two things: either substitute the whole meal with another meal from the same timeband, from another day in the same week (i.e., you can swop any main meal from Days 8–14 with any other main meal from Days 8–14, but not from any other day of the diet). Or you can use the calorie chart at the back of the book to find another food of a similar type which contains roughly the same calories. For example, if 100 g (4 oz) tuna in brine is listed and you don't like tuna, you could swop it for 75 g (3 oz) of drained pink salmon or sardines in brine.

But bear in mind that I have worked out this diet to be nutritionally balanced and to give precise energy levels, so only swop if you have a genuine reason. However, although it is always better to eat what is stated, I'd rather you make an occasional swop than give up on the programme!

• Plan ahead. Make lists and buy what you need in advance.

• Store fresh fruit and vegetables in cool conditions to retain their maximum vitamin content.

Unlimiteds

The following foods and drink may be consumed in unlimited quantities throughout the 21-day schedule:

Water. Drink as much water as you can, to a maximum of 6 glasses a day, especially with meals.

Weak tea or coffee. You may use milk from your daily allowance, except on Days 1 and 2.

Lemon juice.

Fresh or dried herbs and spices.

Tomato purée.

Herbal and fruit teas.

Salad greens, e.g., lettuce, cress and cucumber.

You may also have an occasional calorie-free soft drink, e.g., diet cola, and you may use artificial sweeteners, although I would prefer you to wean yourself off the need for a sweet taste in tea, coffee, etc.

Fruit choices

When the diet states 'C-rich fruit choice', you may choose one of the following:

1 orange
1/2 grapefruit
2 tangerines (or satsumas or similar)
1 kiwifruit
1 x 140–175 g (5–6 oz) serving fresh strawberries or raspberries
1 x 140–200 g (5–7 oz) portion melon

When the diet states 'fruit choice', you may choose one of the following:

1 apple
1 small banana
1 pear
1 peach
1 nectarine
2 fresh apricots
1 or 2 slices of fresh pineapple
1 x 110 g (4 oz) serving grapes
2 dessert plums

When selecting your fruit choices, vary them as much as possible since the nutrient content (e.g., vitamins, fibre) varies from fruit to fruit.

Finally ...

It is best to begin the 21-day schedule on a Saturday so that your 'tough start' falls on two days when you can relax. If, however, Saturday and Sunday are not your days off, start the diet when you do plan to have two 'easy' days.

It is always advisable to check with your doctor before beginning any diet plan. If you are already on any special diet plan given you by your doctor, or suffer from any particular medical condition, it is vital that you show your doctor this plan, and get his or her permission to start.

—— THE ACTIVITY PROGRAMME ——

The activity schedule varies from day to day, becoming progressively more advanced; but, it is always based upon the information and workouts given in Chapters 2–5, and it is important that you read through those chapters before you commence the 21-day programme.

Familiarize yourself with the body contouring and fat burning routines, which everyone will be doing. You may also be undertaking some spot reducing, and you will want to practise some of the ideas you will learn in Chapter 5 on instant slimming and body awareness.

Here is a more detailed analysis of what these four programmes will do for you, but, remember, on each day of the 21-day schedule you must read Your Activities for Today for the. day's relevant programme. This outlines one of a variety of combinations of the workouts on offer.

Never do more than the suggested routines. If you haven't exercised in a while, this could lead to fatigue and/or muscle strain or even injury. If you can't manage the complete routines at first, just follow the advice given at the start of the activity chapters. Be sensible, and read all the instructions within Chapters 2–5 until you know them well.

19

Body Contouring Programme

This programme takes approximately 20 minutes to complete and you will be doing it up to five times a week throughout the 21 days. It is the core of your activity programme and I have designed it specially to work on the body areas that make the most difference to your vital statistics – bust and back, waist and stomach, hips and bottom. The contouring programme alone will not slim you, but it will re-shape your body so that you keep your curves while the diet helps you to lose weight.

The complete contouring programme is explained and illustrated in Chapter 2.

Spot Reducing Programme

In addition to the contouring programme, many of you will also want to do the shorter spot reducing programme. This is simply five minutes or so of exercise concentrated on your own personal problem area – the part of your body that you feel needs most attention.

There are four mini-programmes covering four body areas: bust, chest and upper back; stomach and waist; bottom; hips and thighs.

The spot reducing routines are detailed in Chapter 3. Look at your body, read the chapter and decide whether you want to add one or more of these routines to your 21-day schedule. If the answer is yes, do the routine(s) on the days specified within the schedule, outlined later in this chapter.

Fat Burning Programme

This programme helps you slim down by literally burning up the fat on your body for energy, through a low-intensity aerobic workout. You will all be doing the fat burning programme at least five days a week, starting at 20 minutes per day and gradually building up over the weeks. This programme has the added advantage of helping to burn fat off the most stubborn areas – usually your stomach, bottom, hips and thighs, where women's bodies have a natural tendency to store fat. The intensive lower body workout in this fat burning programme will help to mobilize the fat in these areas.

You'll need no special equipment for the fat burning programme as it is based on aerobic walking – or alternative activities for those times when you can't walk. The full programme is explained in Chapter 4.

On days when you do a fat burning programme and a body contouring programme, try to space them at opposite ends of the day, or at least leave a gap of a few hours between them. Apart from that, it is up to you when you do the programmes during the day.

Instant Slimming Programme

If you want to look, and measure, up to an inch (2.5 cm) slimmer instantly, the programme of body awareness and body re-alignment in Chapter 5 will help you to do just that. Body awareness teaches you to continue the good work that the contouring routine is doing for your body all day through, so that you don't just exercise for half an hour a day then ignore what your body is doing for the other 23^1/$_2$ hours!

If your poor shape is caused by bad posture habits and alignment, this is one programme you really need. Read the chapter, then throughout the 21-day schedule follow the tips given for body awareness and see surprisingly rapid improvements in the way you look.

Short or tall?

For most women of average height, I consider that size 12 is a reasonable target dress size to aim for. By average height, I mean between 5 ft 3 ins (1.6 m) and 5 ft 7 ins (1.7 m).

But, if you happen to be shorter or taller than average, it may be better for you to aim for a different size. If you're small, you may still feel over-curvy at size 12 and want to get down to a 10. If you're very tall, you may find size 12 would leave you too thin, so aim for a 14.

The principles of this diet and activity programme are the same, but here are some special notes for you.

• *If you want to be a size 10*
If you're of petite build and aiming for a size 10, then you may find that following the size-12 diet might take you a little longer to lose the weight you need to lose, although the activity programme will have you shaping up just as quickly as everyone else. This is because shorter people normally need fewer calories than taller people (a short body needs less energy than a tall body to do the same work) and their metabolic rate is slower. So simply repeat the 21-day schedule until you do get there.

• *If you want to be a size 14*
If you are a taller, bigger-boned person you may find that you lose weight more quickly on the size-12 diet. That is because tall people can eat more than average, and have a faster metabolic rate. If this happens to you, or if you feel hungry on the diet, you should simply increase your portion sizes of all the following foods by

25 per cent: bread, potatoes, rice, pasta, and cereals. These high-carbohydrate, low-fat foods will help you to feel full without damaging your weight loss progress.

You too will find the activity programme works just as well for you as for everyone else.

Right, as soon as you have completed your food shopping and read Chapters 2–5, you're all set to begin the 21-day schedule. Remember: give it your best effort and it will work for you.

—WHEN YOUR 21 DAYS ARE OVER—

When you have completed the schedule, most of you will want to go straight on to a maintenance diet and activity programme. These are contained in Chapter 6; they'll help you to stay slim and shapely for the rest of your life.

However, if you came to the programme needing to lose more than one or two dress sizes, you can, if you wish, repeat the whole programme until you are down to your target size. It is perfectly safe for the long term.

There is one important point I must mention about weight loss. If you are a reasonable weight but your figure still needs work, then whatever you do, don't try low-calorie dieting to achieve the shape you want. All you will do is end up being too thin, with no curves, and bags and sags in the wrong places!

What you do need to do is go on to the maintenance diet, outlined in Chapter 6, but continue with the full activity programme described in the 21-day schedule until you have achieved your optimum body shape. Then you can carry on and follow the maintenance activity programme in Chapter 6.

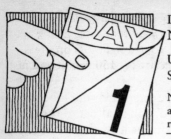

DAILY ALLOWANCES
None.

UNLIMITEDS
See page 17.

Note: Any food listed with an asterisk * has an accompanying recipe.

TODAY I WEIGH
_____stone_____lbs (_____kg)

TODAY I MEASURE
Bust:_____Waist:_____Stomach:_____Hips:_____

Today is the first day of your two-day 'tough start' – a great beginning both for inch and weight loss, and for your motivation.

—— DIET——

On rising
• 75 ml (3 fl oz) unsweet-ened orange juice, plus 1 x 200 ml (7 fl oz, 1/3 pint) glass of mineral water

Breakfast
• 1 apple, including skin
• 1 individual diet fromage frais, any flavour

Mid-morning
• 1 medium banana
• 1 x 200 ml (7 fl oz, 1/3 pint) glass of mineral water

Lunch
• 1 serving Salad Bowl*
• 100 ml (31/2 fl oz) skimmed milk

Mid-afternoon
• 1 diet fruit yogurt, any flavour
• 1 x 200 ml (7 fl oz, 1/3 pint) glass of mineral water

Evening
• 1 serving Salad Bowl*

——RECIPE——

Salad Bowl

Makes 2 servings of approximately 150 calories each

- 100 g (3¹/₂ oz) Iceberg lettuce, sliced
- 2 tender sticks celery, chopped
- 4 radishes, sliced
- 1 small red pepper, de-seeded and sliced
- 50 g (2 oz) cucumber, chopped
- 75 g (3 oz) white grapes, de-seeded and halved or
1 dessert apple, chopped and tossed in lemon juice to
prevent browning
- 50 g (2 oz) cooked chicken (no skin), sliced
- 25 g (1 oz) reduced-fat Cheddar-style cheese, cut into
small cubes
- A little oil-free French dressing (e.g., Waistline)

In a large bowl, combine all the salad and fruit ingredients. Divide the mixture into two. Add the chicken to one and the cheese to the other.

Eat one salad at lunchtime and the other in the evening, adding the oil-free dressing just before serving.

TIPS • You can drink as much water as you like – it'll help you to feel full, and aid your digestion.
• Another feel-full tip is to chew your food well, and eat slowly. • Keep your Salad Bowl meals covered and refrigerated until you're ready to eat them. • Take full advantage of the 'detox diet' on Days 1 and 2 by trying to avoid caffeine-laden tea and coffee. Try a fruit tea instead for a refreshing change. • Do make sure to drink enough throughout these first two days.

——YOUR ACTIVITIES FOR TODAY——

Body Contouring

Familiarize yourself with the complete routine. Run through it slowly, taking your time. The first few attempts will likely take longer than the 20 minutes it will eventually take. Make sure you are doing the moves correctly.

Spot Reducing

No spot reducing programme today; but, if you haven't already done so, read through Chapter 3 and decide whether or not you do need extra work on any of the four spot reduction areas. These are: bust and back; stomach and waist; bottom; hips and thighs.

Fat Burning

No fat burning programme today, but read through Chapter 4 and check you have suitable shoes and clothes for your aerobic walking programme. We'll be starting on Day 2.

Body Awareness and Tips

Introduce yourself to the body awareness and instant slimming tips in Chapter 5. Assess your body in front of a mirror, as described on page 192, and decide whether you need to do the extra exercises outlined within that chapter. Practise a standing pelvic tilt (see page 198). See how much slimmer you look when you stand correctly!

Make sure your mirror is positioned correctly so that you can see your whole body – from top to toe – in one glance.

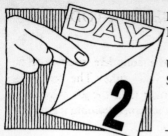

DAILY ALLOWANCES
None.

UNLIMITEDS
See page 17.

Your second, and last, 'tough start' day. Relax and enjoy it!

—— DIET——

On rising
• As Day 1. Try mixing sparkling mineral water with the orange juice, rather than drinking them separately.

Breakfast
• 25 g (1 oz) branflakes with 75 ml (3 fl oz) skimmed milk

Mid-morning
• 1 medium banana
• 1 x 200 ml (7 fl oz, 1/3 pint) glass of mineral water

Lunch
• 1 serving Fruit Bowl*
• 50 ml (2 oz, 2 heaped tablespoons) low-fat natural yogurt

Mid-afternoon
• 25 g (1 oz) reduced-fat Cheddar-style cheese
• 1 x 200 ml (7 fl oz, 1/3 pint) glass of mineral water

Evening
• 1 serving Fruit Bowl*
• 50 ml (2 fl oz, 2 heaped tablespoons) low-fat natural yogurt

——RECIPE——

Fruit Bowl

Makes 2 servings of approximately 115 calories each

- 1 large, juicy orange
- 1 sweet red apple
- 110 g (4 oz) seedless white grapes or soft fruit of choice or melon (weight without skin)
- 1 ripe peach or nectarine or pear
- 2 good teaspoons runny honey
- 1 dessertspoon lemon juice
- Few branflakes

Peel the orange, removing pith, and slice it into segments. Core and chop the apple and add it to the orange in a bowl, stirring well. Halve grapes (or slice soft fruit or melon if using) and add to bowl. Finally, peel peach (or nectarine or pear), chop and add.

Mix honey with the lemon juice and add to bowl, stirring well. You can also add a little water if the fruit hasn't made much of its own juice. Leave for an hour or two so that the flavours mingle.

Eat half at lunchtime and half in the evening, sprinkling with a few branflakes before serving.

——YOUR ACTIVITIES FOR TODAY——

Body Contouring

No body contouring today.

Spot Reducing

Run through your chosen routine (if you have decided to do one). Add it on to the end of your fat burning programme so that your body is already warmed up.

Fat Burning

Today you begin your fat burning programme. Make sure you have read all the instructions in Chapter 4.

Now walk for 20 minutes. Make 5 minutes in the middle of this walk as brisk as you can, following the guidelines for low-intensity aerobic work in Chapter 4.

Aim to cover: 1 mile.

Body Awareness and Tips

Don't forget that your age and current fitness level will have a bearing on how far you can walk in the allotted time. Distances given are only a guide. The younger and/or fitter you are, the further you will walk while keeping your pulse rate in the recommended 60–70 per cent band (see page 169).

TIPS • What time you eat your meals isn't crucial to the programme, but it is usually best to space the meals out evenly and have your evening meal around 7 p.m. If you eat much earlier you may feel hungry at bedtime, which isn't a good idea. If you have to eat your Fruit Bowl early, nibble on some raw carrot or some salad greens later in the evening. And remember, tomorrow you will be feasting!

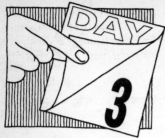

DAILY ALLOWANCES
275 ml (10 fl oz, 1/2 pint)
skimmed milk

UNLIMITEDS
See page 17.

Congratulations! You have made it through the 'tough start'. Now we begin five days of real work on your body. You'll be eating plenty of carbohydrates and really getting 'stuck in' to your activities.

—— DIET——

Breakfast
• 140 ml (5 fl oz, 1/4 pint) unsweetened orange juice or
• 1 C-rich fruit choice (see page 18)
• 25 g (1 oz) branflakes, Bran buds or Fruit 'n' Fibre, with milk from your daily allowance

Mid-morning
• 1 fruit choice (see page 18)

Lunch
• 1 egg and salad sandwich: Use 1 medium (size 3) hard-boiled egg, sliced, with unlimited green salad items plus a sliced tomato. Using medium sliced wholemeal bread, spread 2 slices with a little low-fat spread, fill with egg and salad, and top with 1 level dessertspoon of reduced-calorie mayonnaise or salad cream.
Homemade sandwiches are preferable, but you can substitute a takeaway sandwich without added mayonnaise and on wholemeal bread.

Mid-afternoon
• 1 sachet instant low-calorie soup, plus 1 Ryvita, dark rye or oatbran variety

Evening
• 1 serving of Thai Chicken and Noodle Stir-Fry* OR
• 1 average chicken breast

30

fillet – skinned and brushed with a little low-fat spread or Hoisin sauce, and baked, grilled or microwaved. Serve with 150 g (6 oz) boiled potatoes or rice and 50 g (2 oz) peas (fresh or frozen).
• 1 diet fromage frais, any flavour, with either selection

——RECIPE——

Thai Chicken and Noodle Stir-Fry

Serves 2 at approximately 410 calories per portion

• 1 level dessertspoon runny honey
• 1 level teaspoon brown sugar
• 2 teaspoons lemon juice
• 1 dessertspoon dry or medium sherry
• 1 teaspoon soya sauce
• 1 level teaspoon Thai 7-Spice seasoning
• 100 ml (3½ fl oz) chicken stock from cube, or homemade
• 1 dessertspoon corn or sunflower oil
• 225 g (8 oz) skinned chicken breast fillets, sliced into thin strips
• 1 small onion, sliced thinly
• 1 red pepper, de-seeded and cut into strips
• 1 garlic clove, crushed or ½ teaspoon garlic purée (optional)
• 100 g (3½ oz) fresh beansprouts
• 1 teaspoon cornflour blended with a little cold water
• 110 g (4 oz) medium noodles, cooked according to packet (usually simply soaked in boiling water for a few minutes)

In a small jug or bowl, mix together the honey, sugar, lemon juice, sherry, soya sauce, 7-Spice seasoning and stock. Stir well.

Heat the oil in a medium non-stick pan and add the chicken and onion, stir-frying for a few minutes over a fairly hot heat until chicken is golden.

Add red pepper and garlic, if used, and stir-fry for a further two minutes; add beansprouts and stir-fry for 1 minute.

Add the stock mixture, lower heat and simmer for 2 minutes. Add cornflour mixture and stir to thicken sauce.

Toss noodles in the stir-fry for a few seconds and serve.

TIPS • Thai 7-Spice seasoning is available from most supermarkets and delicatessens. Schwartz do a good one. If you can't find it, though, use 5-Spice seasoning. • Hoisin sauce is a delicious barbecue-type sauce. Alternatively, you could simply brush on a mixture of soya sauce and honey.

——YOUR ACTIVITIES FOR TODAY——

Body Contouring

Do the complete contouring routine today: one set of each exercise. (If you can't manage a complete set of any of the exercises, don't worry – just do what you can and build up.) Do give it your best effort!

Spot Reducing

No spot reducing today.

Fat Burning

Walk for 20 minutes. Make the middle 10 minutes a brisk walk.

Aim to cover: 1 mile plus.

Body Awareness and Tips

Practise the standing pelvic tilt again, and the sitting pelvic tilt (turn to page 198 for details).

Remember, if for some reason you can't do your fat burning walk on any specified day, choose one of the aerobic alternatives in Chapter 4.

TIPS • Don't forget to drink plenty. Water is the preferred drink, but if you like tea and coffee, limit them to around four cups a day, or try decaffeinated. For your health's sake it is better to limit your caffeine intake. • At the end of the day, if there is any milk left over from your daily allowance, use it as a drink on its own.

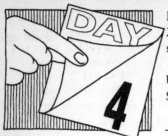

DAILY ALLOWANCES
275 ml (10 fl oz, 1/2 pint)
skimmed milk

UNLIMITEDS
See page 17.

You will be feeling full of vitality now and looking forward to the rest of the programme. Don't forget to plan ahead with your shopping!

—— DIET——

Breakfast
• 1 x 125 g (4 1/2 oz) tub diet fruit yogurt or 2 tablespoons (50 ml, 2 fl oz) low-fat natural yogurt, mixed with 15 g (1/2 oz) branflakes or no-added-sugar muesli and 1 dessert apple, chopped

Mid-morning
• 1 Ryvita, dark rye or oatbran, with a little low-fat spread and Marmite

Lunch
• Beans on toast: 2 slices wholemeal bread from a large, medium-cut loaf, toasted and topped with 1 x 225 g (8 oz) can baked beans in tomato sauce; OR
• 1 Greek-style pitta: Split 1 wholemeal pitta and fill with

1 small (110 g, 4 oz) carton natural low-fat cottage cheese plus chopped green pepper, Iceberg lettuce, spring onion, cucumber, tomato and a couple of black stoned olives (optional). Drizzle oil-free French dressing over and serve.
• 1 C-rich fruit choice (see page 18) with either selection

Mid-afternoon
• 1 fruit choice (see page 18)

Evening
• 1 serving of Tuna and Sweetcorn Jacket Potatoes* with a side salad consisting of any salad greens plus chopped tomato; OR

• 1 Spanish-style omelette: Beat together 2 medium (size 3) eggs with a little seasoning to taste and a dash of cold water. Add 50 g (2 oz) cooked diced potato and 25 g (1 oz) cooked peas. Heat 15 g ($\frac{1}{2}$ oz) low-fat spread in a frying pan; add egg mixture and cook until bottom is golden. Turn over and cook other side. Serve with a 40 g ($1\frac{1}{2}$ oz) piece wholemeal bread and side salad as above.

——RECIPE——

Tuna and Sweetcorn Jacket Potatoes

Serves 2 at approximately 385 calories per portion

• 2 x 275 g (10 oz) baking potatoes
• 50 g (2 oz) whole French beans, cooked and cut in half
• 40 g ($1\frac{1}{2}$ oz) sweetcorn kernels
• 1 x 200 g (7 oz) can tuna in brine, drained
• 50 g (2 oz, 2 good tablespoons) Greek-style or whole-milk yogurt
• A little salt and pepper to taste

Scrub and prick the potatoes and bake them at 200°C (400°F) for approximately 1 hour, until cooked through.

If using frozen sweetcorn kernels, boil them for a few minutes. If using canned, drain. Mix corn with beans, tuna and half the yogurt.

Cut tops off potatoes and scoop out flesh, mash with remaining yogurt and seasoning.

Pile back into potato skins and top with tuna and sweetcorn mixture. The potatoes can be kept and reheated later if necessary, either in the oven for 15 minutes or in a microwave on full for $1\frac{1}{2}$ minutes.

TIPS • Try to cut down on the amount of salt you add to your recipes and at the table. Salt tends to make you retain more fluid, especially around the stomach area. Try a salt substitute instead, such as Lo Salt, if you like. • Your Spanish omelette can be made using finely chopped onion or sweetcorn – or even mushrooms – instead of peas.

——YOUR ACTIVITIES FOR TODAY——

Body Contouring

No body contouring today.

Spot Reducing

Add your chosen spot reducing routine on to the end of today's fat burning programme.

Fat Burning

Walk for 25 minutes. Make the middle 15 minutes a brisk walk.

Aim to cover: 1^1/$_2$ miles.

Body Awareness and Tips

If you decided that you need the extra body re-alignment exercise programme in Chapter 5, today make a start on it (see page 201). Ten minutes is all you need.

When you're walking remember to keep the pelvis tilted correctly, and to walk from the hips.

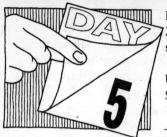

DAILY ALLOWANCES
275 ml (10 fl oz, $^1/_2$ pint)
skimmed milk

UNLIMITEDS
See page 17.

You've completed nearly a quarter of the schedule, so keep thinking positively and picture yourself wearing that size-12 dress within weeks!

—— DIET——

Breakfast
• 40 g (1$^1/_2$ oz) no-added-sugar muesli, with milk from allowance
• 140 ml (5 fl oz, $^1/_4$ pint) unsweetened orange juice or 1 C-rich fruit choice (see page 18)

Mid-morning
• 1 fruit choice (see page 18)

Lunch
• Sandwich: 50 g (2 oz) extra-lean ham or roast turkey or roast beef (all visible fat removed), plus unlimited green salad items and tomatoes in 2 slices of wholemeal bread from a large, medium-sliced loaf. Spread the bread very thinly with low-fat spread and add a teaspoon of mustard or horseradish sauce to taste.
• 1 diet fromage frais, any flavour

Mid-afternoon
• 1 fruit choice (see page 18)

Evening
• 1 serving Cheesy-Topped Fish* with 150 g (6 oz) new or boiled potatoes and 110 g (4 oz) broccoli; OR
• 1 x 175 g (6 oz) white fish fillet of your choice, plain-grilled, baked or micro-waved with potatoes and broccoli as above; plus 50 g (2 oz) vanilla ice cream or 1 French-style set fruit yogurt

—— RECIPE——

Cheesy-Topped Fish

Serves 2 at approximately 265 calories per portion

• 2 x 175 g (6 oz) white fish fillets; e.g., cod, coley, plaice or haddock
• 1 dessertspoon olive or corn oil
• 1 medium tomato, de-seeded and chopped small
• 2 spring onions, chopped
• 25 g (1 oz) reduced-fat Cheddar-style cheese, grated
• 2 level tablespoons reduced-calorie mayonnaise
• Seasoning to taste

Brush the fish fillets with the oil and, depending on thickness, grill under a fairly hot heat for 3–4 minutes, turning if necessary.

Meanwhile, mix together all the remaining ingredients, cover the top of the fish portions with it and grill until the cheesy mixture is bubbling – approximately 2 minutes.

——YOUR ACTIVITIES FOR TODAY——

Body Contouring

Do the complete contouring routine today: one set of each exercise. Aching muscles should not be a problem. If you do have any serious aches, be doubly careful about doing the warm-up and cool-down properly, and make sure your room is warm enough while you exercise.

Spot Reducing

Do your chosen spot reducing routine today at the end of your contouring routine.

Fat Burning

No fat burning programme today.

Body Awareness and Tips

How do you walk up stairs? You can burn off some extra calories and improve your calf shape if you glide quickly up stairs placing the ball of each foot lightly on each stair as you go. Don't let your heels touch the stairs at all. When you're fitter, running up stairs is a good way to burn off extra calories.

Don't forget, you can mix and match your spot reducing routines (see page 140).

No fat burning programme today.

TIPS • Throughout the 21 days, there is always at least one lunch suggestion that you can pack and take to work. Usually it is best to take dressings separately and add just before eating to prevent any salad and bread items becoming soggy.

• When sandwich choices are given, like today, it is best to make your own, but you may substitute a take away sandwich of the same kind. It is best if you go to a sandwich bar that will make up your sandwich while you watch so that you can avoid the two things likely to pile on the calories – spreading the bread thickly with butter or margarine, and adding loads of mayonnaise.

• Turkey is the safest filling out of the choices given in today's sandwich for a takeaway lunch, as sandwich-bar ham and beef may be quite fatty.

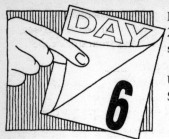

DAILY ALLOWANCES
275 ml (10 fl oz, 1/2 pint)
skimmed milk

UNLIMITEDS
See page 17.

Has anyone noticed how good you're looking yet? If clothes are already far too loose, remember it won't be long before you can treat yourself to one or two new outfits.

—— DIET——

Breakfast
• 1 large banana chopped into 1 small tub of natural low-fat yogurt, with 1 teaspoon honey added

Mid-morning
• 1 Ryvita, dark rye or oatbran, with Marmite; OR
• 1 sachet low-calorie instant soup

Lunch
• 1 ready-made French Bread Pizza, either ham and mushroom, pineapple and ham, or cheese and tomato, served with unlimited green salad items; OR
• Cheese sandwich: Spread 2 slices wholemeal bread (large loaf, medium cut)

with a little low-fat spread. Grate 50 g (2 oz) reduced-fat Cheddar-style cheese and fill sandwich. Top with unlimited green salad items, plus tomatoes and a chopped spring onion.

Mid-afternoon
• 1 C-rich fruit choice (see page 18)

Evening
• 1 serving Paprika Pork* with a green salad and either 140 g (5 oz) instant mashed potato or 75 g (3 oz) boiled rice or noodles; OR
• 110 g (4 oz) tenderloin pork steak or extra-lean pork chop, trimmed of fat, grilled, and served with

175 g (6 oz) baked or boiled potato, 75 g (3 oz) peas and 75 g (3 oz) carrots, plus

either 1 dessertspoon apple sauce or an average serving of gravy from stock cube

——RECIPE——

Paprika Pork

Serves 2 at approximately 290 calories per portion

- 1 tablespoon corn, olive or sunflower oil
- 225 g (8 oz) pork fillet, cubed
- 1 large onion, finely chopped
- 1 clove garlic, crushed (optional)
- 110 g (4 oz) button mushrooms, halved
- 1 heaped dessertspoon paprika
- Pinch ground cumin
- 200 g (7 oz) chopped, canned tomatoes
- 140 ml (5 fl oz, ¼ pint) chicken stock from cube or homemade
- Black pepper and a little salt
- 1 level teaspoon sugar
- Dash lemon juice
- 50 g (2 oz) Greek-style yogurt
- Chopped chives or parsley to garnish

Heat the oil in a non-stick frying pan and brown the pork in it a little at a time; remove from pan.

Add onion and stir-fry over medium heat until soft, adding garlic, if using, towards the end. Add mushrooms and stir again for 2 minutes. Add paprika and cumin and stir well; add tomatoes, stock, seasoning and sugar.

Cover and simmer for approximately 30 minutes or until everything is tender and you have a rich sauce.

To serve, add a dash of lemon juice to the Greek-style yogurt, swirl the yogurt over the pork and top with herbs for garnish.

TIPS • Chicken can be used instead of pork in the recipe dish if you like. • Make a note of recipes and meals you particularly enjoy on the 21-day schedule so that when you switch to the maintenance diet you can try them again. • Fresh herbs can often be kept growing in pots on your windowsill all winter long. Freshly cut herbs store well in the fridge inside plastic bags. • Vegetarians could try Quorn chunks in the paprika casserole, instead of pork.

——YOUR ACTIVITIES FOR TODAY——

Body Contouring

Do the complete contouring programme today and try to speed up the pace a little by putting more effort into the movements (without jerking), and by pausing for less time between exercises.

Spot Reducing

No spot reducing today.

Fat Burning

Walk for 25 minutes. Make the middle 15 minutes of your walk brisk.

Aim to cover: 1½ miles plus.

Body Awareness and Tips

Remember that for quickest body re-alignment you should continuously be aware of how you are using your body all day long. Sit right, stand right, walk right.

Start to think about other activities you could include in your life – how about joining some kind of sports club, or going swimming regularly? Visit your local authority leisure centre for ideas.

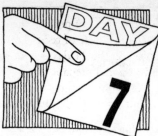

DAILY ALLOWANCES
275 ml (10 fl oz, ¹/₂ pint)
skimmed milk

UNLIMITEDS
See page 17.

This is the last day of your first week, so give yourself a
pat on the back.

—— DIET——

Breakfast
• 140 ml (5 fl oz, ¹/₄ pint)
unsweetened orange juice or
1 C-rich fruit choice (see
page 18)
• 25 g (1 oz) branflakes or
Bran Buds or Fruit 'n' Fibre,
with milk from your daily
allowance

Mid-morning
• 1 fruit choice (see page 18)

Lunch
• Tuna bap: Spread one
large wholemeal bap with a
little low-fat spread, and fill
with 100 g (3¹/₂ oz) tuna in
brine, drained. Top with
sliced tomato, onion rings,
green salad and chopped
parsley and add a few
canned, drained butter
beans. Drizzle on some

oil-free French dressing.
• 1 diet fruit yogurt, any
flavour

Mid-afternoon
• 1 Ryvita, dark rye or
oatbran, with 1 teaspoon
honey

Evening
• 1 serving Indonesian
Turkey with Rice* OR
• 1 average chicken portion,
skinned and brushed with a
mixture of 1 teaspoon olive
oil, 1 teaspoon runny honey,
1 teaspoon lemon juice, a
little garlic purée, and salt
and black pepper. Grill or
bake the chicken until
cooked through. Serve with
225 g (8 oz) baked potato
and 110 g (4 oz) green
beans.

——RECIPE——

Indonesian Turkey with Rice

Serves 2 at approximately 450 calories per portion

- 110 g (4 oz) long-grain rice
- Little salt
- 1 tablespoon corn or sunflower oil
- 175 g (6 oz) turkey (or chicken) fillet, cut into bite-sized pieces
- 1 carrot, peeled and pared into thin slices
- 1 small red pepper, de-seeded and chopped
- 110 g (4 oz) fresh beansprouts
- 4 spring onions, chopped
- 50 g (2 oz) peeled prawns
- $1/2$ teaspoon garlic purée (optional)
- 1 tablespoon soya sauce
- 1 good teaspoon 7-Spice seasoning
- Pinch brown sugar

Cook the rice in boiling water until just tender, with a little salt added, then set aside.

Heat oil in a large non-stick frying pan and stir-fry the turkey over a high heat for a minute to brown. Turn heat down slightly and add carrot and pepper, stir-frying again for approximately 3 minutes.

Add all the remaining ingredients, including the rice, and cook over a medium heat for 2 or 3 minutes, stirring gently all the time. You may add a little chicken stock or water if the mixture seems to be sticking to the pan, or you prefer it slightly less dry.

Taste for seasoning and serve.

> **TIPS** • For vegetarians, tofu, plain or smoked, is
> an acceptable substitute for turkey in the main
> meal recipe. • Basmati rice is the best long-grain
> rice for flavour.

——YOUR ACTIVITIES FOR TODAY——

Body Contouring

No body contouring today.

Spot Reducing

Add your chosen spot reducing programme to your fat
burning programme today.

Fat Burning

Walk for 30 minutes. Warm up for 5 minutes, then
ensure you walk briskly for the next 20. Slow down the
pace for the last 5 minutes.

Aim to cover: 2 miles.

Body Awareness and Tips

Learn to listen to your body telling you how it feels. For
instance, if you feel really good during your fat-burning
walk and would like to stay walking a little longer, then
do. But only maintain the brisk pace for as long as the
schedule tells you.

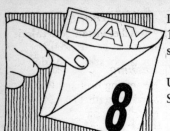

DAILY ALLOWANCES
140 ml (5 fl oz, 1/4 pint)
skimmed milk

UNLIMITEDS
See page 17.

TODAY I WEIGH
_____stone _____lbs(_____ kg)

TODAY I MEASURE
Bust:_____ Waist:_____ Stomach:_____ Hips:_____

I HAVE LOST A TOTAL OF
_____ lbs (_____ kg)

I HAVE LOST A TOTAL OF
_____ ins (_____ cm)

Now we begin the next phase of your 21-day schedule.
We're taking the calories down just a little bit to keep
that fat moving off, and we're really into the swing of
the activity programme now.

—— DIET——

Breakfast
• 25 g (1 oz) branflakes,
with milk from allowance
• 1 C-rich fruit choice (see
page 18)

Mid-morning
• 1 fruit choice (see page 18)

Lunch
• Ploughman's: 50 g (2 oz)
piece French bread
(preferably wholemeal), with
a little low-fat spread; 40 g
(1½ oz) reduced-fat
Cheddar-style cheese; 2
pickled onions (optional),
salad of spring onions,

tomato and lettuce; plus
1 apple; OR
• Cheese on toast: 40 g
(1¹/₂ oz) grated reduced-fat
Cheddar, on 1 slice wholemeal toast from a large
medium-cut loaf, topped
with chopped tomato and
grilled; plus 1 large banana

Mid-afternoon
• 1 sachet instant low calorie
soup

Evening
• 1 serving Beef and Pepper
Stir-Fry* with 110 g (4 oz)
boiled rice; OR
• 1 x 110 g (4 oz) beefburger
made from extra-lean mince,
well-grilled, in 1 wholemeal
bap with a large mixed salad

——RECIPE——

Beef and Pepper Stir-Fry
Serves 2 at approximately 275 calories per portion

• 175 g (6 oz) rump or minute steak, cut into strips
• 1 tablespoon corn, olive or sunflower oil
• 1 red pepper, de-seeded and sliced
• 1 green pepper, de-seeded and sliced
• 4 spring onions, cut into 1-inch lengths
• 1 teaspoon 5-Spice seasoning
• 110 g (4 oz) water chestnuts, halved
• ¹/₂ teaspoon garlic purée (optional)
• 2 tablespoons Hoisin sauce
• Little beef stock from cube

Heat oil in large non-stick frying pan and stir-fry the
beef on a high heat until browned.

Add peppers and cook for a minute then turn heat
down a little, add onions and stir-fry for a few more
minutes.

Add seasoning, chestnuts, garlic and Hoisin sauce and
stir for a further minute.

Add a little beef stock to produce a thick sauce.

TIPS • You can add a knob of peeled fresh ginger to this stir-fry if you like. Add it when you add the peppers, but remove before serving. • For a weight-maintenance diet, you can add some flaked almonds to this dish.

——YOUR ACTIVITIES FOR TODAY——

Body Contouring

You should be noticing a very real improvement in your body shape by now – smaller waist, tighter hips and thighs and a flatter tummy. Do the complete standard routine, but today try to do two sets of at least some of the exercises: those you are beginning to find easiest.

Spot Reducing

No spot reducing today.

Fat Burning

It's the weekend, so let's take another walk today. Walk for 30 minutes. Make the middle 20 minutes brisk.

Aim to cover: 2 miles plus.

Body Awareness and Tips

Start Week 2 by really working on any posture problems. Complete the full body re-alignment exercise set (see page 201).

Did you know that housework is a good suppling and toning exercise? It can burn off quite a few calories, too. See how much effort you can put into those usual chores like bed-making, vacuuming and polishing.

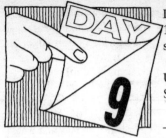

DAILY ALLOWANCES
140 ml (5 fl oz, ¼ pint)
skimmed milk

UNLIMITEDS
See page 17.

You will have noticed that on the 21-day schedule, the diet doesn't allow for 'naughty' treats or extras such as cake or alcohol. That's because this programme requires only one thing from you for it to work: real commitment. Anyone who is determined – and that's you – would like to be shown a pure, healthy, slimming way of eating, to help you to feel healthy and good about yourself. After you finish the schedule, you can introduce 'treats' such as chocolate and wine, as you'll see in Chapter 6. Once you've learnt the basics of a good diet, being sensible about those extras will be easier.

—— DIET——

Breakfast
• 25 g (1 oz, 1 slice from large medium-cut loaf) wholemeal bread with a little low-fat spread and 2 teaspoons pure fruit spread
• 1 x 140 ml (5 fl oz, ¼ pint) glass unsweetened orange juice or 1 C-rich fruit choice (see page 18)

Mid-morning
• 1 diet fruit yogurt, any flavour

Lunch
• Tuna pitta: Fill 1 whole-wheat pitta with 1 x 100 g (3½ oz) can of tuna in brine, drained and flaked, plus 1 serving of homemade Coleslaw* and sliced tomato; OR

• Tuna sandwich: 2 slices of wholemeal bread from a large medium-cut leaf, with a little low-fat spread and filled with tuna, coleslaw and tomato as above

Mid-afternoon
• 1 fruit choice (see page 18)

Evening
• 1 serving No-Meat Bolognese* with 125 g (4½ oz) boiled spaghetti (preferably wholewheat) served with a green salad; OR
• 100 g (3½ oz) roast chicken (no skin) served with 110 g (4 oz) boiled potatoes, 75 g (3 oz) peas or sweetcorn, 110 g (4 oz) carrots or cabbage and a little gravy from stock cube (no added fat)

——RECIPES——

Coleslaw
Serves 2 at approximately 60 calories per portion

• 1 good tablespoon low-fat natural yogurt
• 1 level tablespoon reduced-calorie mayonnaise
• 1 teaspoon lemon juice
• Salt and black pepper to taste
• 110 g (4 oz) white cabbage, finely sliced
• 50 g (2 oz) carrot, grated
• 25 g (1 oz) onion, very finely chopped
• 15 g (1 oz) sultanas

Beat the yogurt together with the mayonnaise, lemon juice and seasoning. Add rest of ingredients and mix well before serving.

No-Meat Bolognese

Serves 2 at approximately 260 calories per portion

- 75 g (3 oz) brown lentils
- 1 tablespoon corn, olive or sunflower oil
- 1 large onion, finely chopped
- 1 clove garlic, crushed
- 1 large stick celery, finely chopped
- 50 g (2 oz) mushrooms, sliced
- 1 small carrot, grated
- 1 x 200 g (7 oz) can chopped tomatoes
- 1 bay leaf (optional)
- Little salt and black pepper

Boil the lentils in plenty of water for 30–40 minutes, or until soft. Drain, but retain water.

Heat the oil in a non-stick frying pan and stir-fry onion until transparent with a tinge of gold. Add the cooked lentils and stir-fry for 2 minutes.

Add the rest of the ingredients, bring to simmer, stir well, cover and simmer for 30 minutes or so. You may need to add a little of the lentil water (or vegetable stock) towards end of cooking.

Remove bay leaf before serving.

TIPS • For a change, you can use double the mushrooms and omit the carrot from the Bolognese sauce. You could also add a pinch of chilli powder for a spicier flavour. • Don't forget to keep drinking plenty of water, especially at mealtimes. • To save wholemeal pittas becoming dry when you heat them, sprinkle with a little water before warming in the oven for a few minutes.

51

——YOUR ACTIVITIES FOR TODAY——

Body Contouring

Try two complete sets of the standard exercises today.

Spot Reducing

No spot reducing today.

Fat Burning

Walk for 40 minutes. Make 20 of them brisk.
  Aim to cover: 2 miles plus.

Body Awareness and Tips

Concentrate on swinging those arms out when you walk,
and take nice long strides. Breathe in deeply.

  Try to concentrate on your breathing, no matter what
you are doing throughout the day. Remember that the
more oxygen you give your body, the better your metabolism will work and the better it will burn fat.

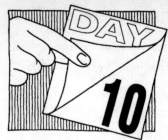

DAILY ALLOWANCES
140 ml (5 fl oz, ¼ pint)
skimmed milk

UNLIMITEDS
See page 17.

Nearly halfway. You're doing really well. Can you feel the difference?

—— DIET——

Breakfast
• 1 x 125 g (4½ oz) tub of natural low-fat yogurt, with 1 small banana, chopped and mixed in

Mid-morning
• 1 C-rich fruit choice (see page 18)

Lunch
• Spicy chicken sandwich: Mix 50 g (2 oz) cooked chopped chicken meat (no skin) with 1 teaspoon reduced-calorie mayonnaise, ½ teaspoon mild curry powder and a dash of lemon juice. Spread 1 slice of wholemeal bread from a large medium-cut loaf with slices of Iceberg lettuce and cucumber, top with the chicken mixture, more lettuce and cucumber, and finish with another slice of bread; plus 50 g (2 oz) grapes or 1 satsuma; OR
• Chicken rice salad: Mix 75 g (3 oz) cooled boiled rice with 50 g (2 oz) cooked chopped chicken and one small handful sultanas. Add a little chopped celery and chopped raw mushrooms and toss in oil-free French dressing; plus 1 fruit choice (see page 18)

Mid-afternoon
• 1 sachet low-calorie instant soup

Evening
• 1 serving of Pancakes Oriental* with a large green side salad; OR

53

• 110 g (4 oz) peeled prawns plus a large green salad dressed with 1 teaspoon reduced-calorie mayonnaise mixed with a little tomato purée and a pinch of paprika (optional); 50 g (2 oz) chunk of bread or 2 slices of bread from small medium-cut loaf; plus 1 diet fromage frais, any flavour

——RECIPE——

Pancakes Oriental

Serves 2 at approximately 345 calories per portion

• 1 level dessertspoon corn or sunflower oil
• 50 g (2 oz) diced tofu or cooked chicken (no skin)
• 2 spring onions, chopped
• 1 small green pepper, de-seeded and chopped
• 1/2 teaspoon garlic purée (optional)
• 50 g (2 oz) beansprouts
• 2 teaspoons soya sauce
• 2 tablespoons Hoisin or Sweet and Sour sauce
• 100 g (3 1/2 oz) peeled prawns
• 4 ready-prepared crêpes (or use Basic Pancake Recipe, page 55)

Heat oil in a non-stick frying pan and stir-fry the tofu or chicken until golden.

Add onions and pepper and cook for further 3 minutes until soft.

Add garlic (if used), beansprouts, sauces and prawns and stir over medium heat for a further minute.

Divide mixture between crêpes and roll up. Warm for a few minutes in a medium oven, or for 1 minute in a microwave.

TIPS • Ready-prepared crêpes can be purchased at most supermarkets – you'll find them near the pre-packaged breads. If you make your own, following the Basic Pancake Recipe below, the calorie count will not be much different. • If you can find bottled plum sauce, it makes a nice alternative to the Hoisin or Sweet and Sour sauce in the recipe.

Basic Pancake Recipe

Makes 4 pancakes at 120 calories each or 5 at 100 calories each

• 80 g (3 oz) plain flour, sifted with a pinch of salt
• 50 ml (2 fl oz) water mixed with 80 ml (3 fl oz) skimmed milk
• 1 small (size 4) egg
• 10 g (1/3 oz) butter

Beat all the ingredients except butter together in a bowl until smooth.

Melt a little of the butter in a heavy-based small frying pan and tip pan round to coat the bottom. When the fat is very hot, add 2–3 tablespoons of the batter, swirl it around and cook until underside is golden (about 1 minute). When one pancake is cooked, turn it out and keep warm.

Heat pan again and add more mixture, and carry on until you have made all the pancakes, adding the remaining butter when the pan gets very dry. However, in a non-stick pan you should hardly need any butter once the pan gets really hot.

For thin pancakes like these, you don't need to turn them. If rolling them round a filling, make sure the golden side is on the outside.

Note: The calories in the Pancakes Oriental recipe have been calculated on the basis of using pancakes at 100 calories each.

——YOUR ACTIVITIES FOR TODAY——

Body Contouring

Do two standard sets today.

Spot Reducing

Do your chosen spot reducing programme today. Add it on to the end of the contouring programme.

Fat Burning

No fat burning today.

Body Awareness and Tips

Translate many of the moves you do during your contouring routine into everyday life. For instance, while waiting for a kettle to boil or while waiting for the copier at the office, practise your pelvic tilt; do some triceps stretches and calf lifts. Every little bit helps and even a surreptitious movement is better than just standing around. Doing something will make you feel more positive, too.

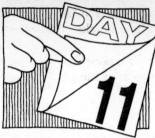

DAILY ALLOWANCES
140 ml (5 fl oz, ¼ pint)
skimmed milk

UNLIMITEDS
See page 17.

You're past the halfway stage now; keep confident and keep working.

—— DIET——

Breakfast
• 25 g (1 oz) branflakes, Bran Buds or Fruit 'n' Fibre with milk from allowance, plus 1 fruit choice (see page 18), chopped or mixed in

Mid-morning
• 1 C-rich fruit choice (see page 18)

Lunch
• 1 sachet low-calorie instant soup
• 2 Ryvitas, dark rye or oatbran, spread with a little low-fat spread and topped with 100 g (3½ oz) pink salmon or 50 g (2 oz) Philadelphia Light, plus sliced cucumber and a side salad of lettuce, cress and onion (or similar)

Mid-afternoon
• 1 diet fromage frais, any flavour

Evening
1 serving Cheesy Baked Potatoes* with a large mixed salad; OR
• 1 x 275 g (10 oz) baked potato, plus 75 g (3 oz) baked beans and 1 serving homemade Coleslaw (see recipe, page 50) or 100 g (3½ oz) commercial diet coleslaw

——RECIPE——

Cheesy Baked Potatoes

Serves 2 at approximately 365 calories per portion

- 2 x 225 g (8 oz) baking potatoes
- 4 tablespoons skimmed milk
- 15 g (½ oz) low-fat spread
- 2 tablespoons beaten egg
- 4 finely-chopped spring onions or 1 small onion, chopped
- 50 g (2 oz) reduced-fat Cheddar-style cheese, grated
- Pinch of chilli powder
- Sprig parsley, chopped, to garnish

Scrub and prick the potatoes, and bake them at 200°C (400°F) for 1 hour or until soft.

Cut tops off and scoop out flesh; mash potato with the milk, low-fat spread and egg and add the onion, cheese, chilli and a little seasoning if required.

Pile mixture into potato cases and reheat for a few minutes. Sprinkle on parsley to serve.

TIPS • If you prefer, you can cook your baked potatoes in the microwave, on full power for about 10 minutes, for two. To help the skins become crispy, wrap the potatoes in kitchen paper. • Chopped chives can also be used to garnish baked, filled potatoes.

——YOUR ACTIVITIES FOR TODAY——

Body Contouring
No body contouring today.

Spot Reducing
Do your chosen spot reducing routine at the end of the fat burning programme.

Fat Burning
Today walk for 40 minutes. Make 25 minutes of your walk brisk.

Aim to cover: 2$^{1}/_{2}$ miles plus.

Body Awareness and Tips
If you decided to carry out the 10-minute body re-alignment programme, today is the day to do it. Make sure you concentrate hard on the moves to get the most from your body without straining it.

Are you training yourself to break the habit of bending over to read books and magazines? Hold the book up in front of you. If you need to get too close, check that your eyesight is all right. When you hunch over, your lungs are compressed and you won't be breathing in all that lovely oxygen!

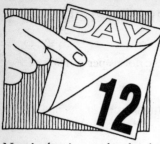

DAILY ALLOWANCES
140 ml (5 fl oz, 1/4 pint)
skimmed milk

UNLIMITEDS
See page 17.

Now's the time to book a hairdressing appointment, or even treat yourself to a make-up lesson, so that your hair and face do justice to your emerging new figure!

—— DIET——

Breakfast
• 1 x 125 g (4½ oz) tub natural low-fat yogurt, topped with a handful (about 15 g, ½ oz) of no-added-sugar muesli and 1 level teaspoon of runny honey

Mid-morning
• C-rich fruit choice (see page 18)

Lunch
• 1 serving Spanish Eggs with Peppers* plus 1 slice wholemeal toast from a large, medium-sliced loaf; OR
• Egg and salad sandwich (see Day 3, page 30)

Mid-afternoon
• 1 fruit choice (see page 18)

Evening
• 1 serving Pasta Twists with Tuna and Tomato* plus a green side salad; OR
• A frozen or chilled ready-prepared single-serving meal of your choice, based on pasta, to a maximum of 350 calories – e.g., Healthy Options Vegetable Lasagne, Marks and Spencer Tagliatelle, or Tesco Spaghetti Bolognese. Serve with a side salad.

Day 12

——RECIPES——

Spanish Eggs with Peppers
Serves 2 at approximately 190 calories per portion

- 1 tablespoon olive oil
- 1 small onion, sliced very thinly
- 1 clove garlic, crushed (optional)
- 1 large green pepper, de-seeded and sliced
- 1 large red pepper, de-seeded and sliced
- Salt to taste
- Dash unsweetened orange juice
- 2 large (size 2) eggs
- 1 level teaspoon sweet paprika

Heat oil in non-stick frying pan and sauté onion until soft.

Add garlic (if used) and peppers and continue sautéing until onion is golden and peppers are soft and slightly brown at edges.

Add salt and orange juice, cover and simmer for 10–15 minutes.

Poach the eggs. Divide pepper mixture between two gratin dishes, making a well in the middle.

Slide eggs into centre and serve with a little paprika sprinkled over.

61

Pasta Twists with Tuna and Tomato

Serves 2 at approximately 370 calories per portion

- 1 tablespoon olive oil
- 1 medium onion, finely chopped
- 50 ml (2 fl oz) dry white wine
- 1 x 200 g (7 oz) can chopped tomatoes with herbs
- 1 level dessertspoon tomato purée
- 110 g (4 oz) pasta twists or other shape
- 1 x 185 g (6 oz) can tuna in brine, drained
- Little salt and black pepper
- Fresh basil or parsley to garnish

Heat oil in a non-stick frying pan and stir-fry onion until soft and tinged with gold. Add wine and bring to bubble. Add tomatoes and purée and simmer for 10 minutes.

Boil the pasta in plenty of lightly salted water until cooked.

Add tuna to tomato sauce with salt and pepper to taste and mix cooked pasta in with sauce.

Serve garnished with herbs.

TIPS • Add a few chopped button mushrooms to the pasta sauce for a change; they will add hardly any calories. • If chopped tomatoes with herbs aren't available, use plain chopped tomatoes and add 1 level teaspoon mixed Mediterranean herbs, or just plain oregano.

——YOUR ACTIVITIES FOR TODAY——

Body Contouring

Do two complete sets of the standard exercises.

Spot Reducing

Do your chosen spot reducing routine today and add it on to your contouring routine.

Fat Burning

Walk for 40 minutes. Make 25 minutes of the walk brisk.

Aim to cover: 2^{1}/2 miles plus.

Body Awareness and Tips

Check out your body profile in the mirror today and see how it is improving. But don't forget – relax and look at yourself as you are naturally. You should see a big difference between now and when you did this on the first day!

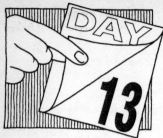

DAILY ALLOWANCES
140 ml (5 fl oz, ¼ pint)
skimmed milk

UNLIMITEDS
See page 17.

As we near the end of the second week, don't flag! If you need motivation just keep looking at all those lovely clothes you'll soon be able to wear. Only two days to weigh and measure day. And you really will be pleased, you can count on that!

—— DIET——

Breakfast
• 1 slice wholemeal bread from a large, medium-cut loaf, with a little low-fat spread and 2 teaspoons pure fruit spread
• 1 x 140 ml (5 fl oz, ¼ pint) glass of unsweetened orange juice or 1 C-rich fruit choice (see page 18)

Mid-morning
• 1 diet fromage frais, any flavour

Lunch
• 1 average pizza slice with unlimited green salad items and tomatoes; plus 1 fruit choice (see page 18); OR
• 1 x 50 g (2 oz) wholemeal roll with a little low-fat spread filled with 50 g (2 oz) Philadelphia Light, plus unlimited green salad items and sliced tomato; plus 1 satsuma or 50 g (2 oz) grapes

Mid-afternoon
• 1 sachet instant low-calorie soup

Evening
• 1 serving Spicy Pork Kebabs* with 125 g (4½ oz) boiled rice and a large mixed salad; OR

• 1 average chicken portion or 100 g (3½ oz) pork tenderloin steak, grilled, served with 1 x 225 g (8 oz)

baked potato and 100 g (3½ oz) peas, sweetcorn or baked beans

——RECIPE——

Spicy Pork Kebabs

Serves 2 at approximately 240 calories per portion

• 1 dessertspoon corn, sunflower or olive oil
• 1 dessertspoon soya sauce
• 1 teaspoon honey
• 1 level teaspoon barbecue seasoning, plus a pinch of chilli
• 2 tablespoons (30 ml, 1 fl oz) orange juice
• 225 g (8 oz) fillet of pork or chicken, cut into bite-sized cubes
• 50 g (2 oz) dried 'no-need-to-soak' apricot halves

Mix together the oil, soya sauce, honey, seasoning and orange juice, pour it over the pork pieces and leave to marinate for at least an hour. (You can leave overnight if you like.)

Thread meat alternately on to skewers with the apricot pieces. Brush with marinade, and grill or barbecue, turning occasionally, until pork is golden and cooked through – about 10 minutes.

Baste from time to time with remaining marinade.

TIPS • Lean fillet of lamb can be used instead of pork or chicken. • Instead of the barbecue seasoning, you can use a level teaspoon of mixed spice made by mixing equal quantities of ground ginger, turmeric and coriander with a pinch of chilli.

——YOUR ACTIVITIES FOR TODAY——

Body Contouring

No body contouring today; take a rest!

Spot Reducing

Do your chosen spot reducing programme after your fat burning exercise.

Fat Burning

Walk 40 minutes today. Make 25 of those brisk.
Aim to cover: 2¹/₂ miles plus.

Body Awareness and Tips

You should be using your walking time not only to get fit and burn off fat, but to relax and enjoy that time to yourself. Remember it is also a good idea to vary your routes so that you don't get bored. By now you can also, if you like, do a little gradient walking – uphill walks will get the fat moving off your bottom, hips and thighs even faster! But count downhill as your cool down towards home.

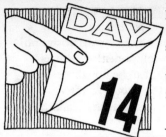

DAILY ALLOWANCES
140 ml (5 fl oz, ¼ pint)
skimmed milk

UNLIMITEDS
See page 17.

Two weeks have flown by, haven't they? Try very hard today because you'll soon be measuring up!

—— DIET——

Breakfast
• 25 g (1 oz) branflakes, Bran Buds or Fruit 'n' Fibre, with milk from your daily allowance
• 1 C-rich fruit choice (see page 18)

Mid-morning
• 1 Ryvita, dark rye or oatbran, with a little low-fat spread and Marmite

Lunch
• Ham sandwich: Spread 2 slices of wholemeal bread from a large, medium-cut loaf with a little low-fat spread and fill with 50 g (2 oz) extra-lean ham, plus plenty of green salad items and tomato, mustard if liked, plus 1 tablespoon diet coleslaw or homemade Coleslaw (see recipe on page 50); OR
• 1 large (size 2) egg, poached, on 1 slice of wholemeal toast from a large medium-cut loaf; plus 1 medium banana

Mid-afternoon
• 1 fruit choice (see page 18)

Evening
• 1 serving Seafood Medley* with 140 g (5 oz) boiled rice or potatoes and a green salad; OR
• 175 g (6 oz) white fish fillet, grilled with 1 teaspoon butter brushed on it, and served with 140 g (5 oz) instant mashed potato, 75 g (3 oz) peas and 110 g (4 oz) carrots

> **TIPS** • Don't be afraid to experiment with new herbs and spices. Just use a little to start with until you discover which ones you prefer. • Mussels are a low-calorie treat that can be bought ready-prepared in jars or from the freezer counter.

———RECIPE———

Seafood Medley

Serves 2 at approximately 250 calories per portion

- 1 dessertspoon olive oil
- 1 small onion, finely chopped
- 1 small courgette, sliced
- 1 large green pepper, de-seeded and chopped
- 50 g (2 oz) button mushrooms, sliced
- 200 g (7 oz) chopped, canned tomatoes
- Dash of dry white wine (optional)
- 1/2 teaspoon garlic purée (optional)
- 1 level teaspoon chopped dill weed or basil
- Salt and pepper to taste
- 1 x 175 g (6 oz) monkfish or cod fillet, cubed
- 1 x 175 g (6 oz) plaice or lemon sole fillet, cut into strips
- 50 g (2 oz) peeled prawns or shelled mussels

Heat oil in a large non-stick frying pan and stir-fry the onion until soft and transparent. Add courgettes and peppers and fry until soft.

Add mushrooms and stir for a further minute, then add tomatoes, wine, garlic purée (if used), herbs and seasoning and white fish and simmer for 5–6 minutes.

Stir in prawns or mussels, simmer for 1 minute and serve.

——YOUR ACTIVITIES FOR TODAY——

Body Contouring

Do one set of standard exercises and also try one set (or as much as you can manage) of the super versions.

Spot Reducing

Do your spot reducing programme today at the end of the contouring programme.

Fat Burning

No fat burning today.

Body Awareness and Tips

If you are doing the extra exercises, complete your 10-minute body alignment programme today. Do it at the opposite end of the day from the contouring and don't forget to warm up and cool down.

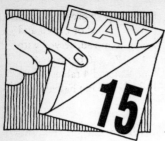

DAILY ALLOWANCES
140 ml (5 fl oz, 1/4 pint) skimmed milk

UNLIMITEDS
See page 17.

TODAY I WEIGH
_____ stone _____ lbs (_____ kg)

TODAY I MEASURE
Bust:_____ Waist:_____ Stomach_____ Hips:_____

I HAVE LOST A TOTAL OF
_____ lbs (_____ kg)

I HAVE LOST A TOTAL OF
_____ ins (_____ cm)

It's downhill all the way from here. Just one week to that size-12 dress! This week's diet is packed full of super-carbohydrates, fruit and vegetables to help you slim off the last few pounds easily. The activity programme hots up even more, and I guarantee you'll enjoy it.

—— DIET——

Breakfast
• 1 diet fromage frais, any flavour
• 1 C-rich fruit choice (see page 18)

Mid-morning
• 1 x 275 ml (10 fl oz, 1/2 pint) glass of mineral water

Lunch
• 1 x 50 g (2 oz) wholemeal bap with a very little low-fat spread and filled with 1 x 110 g (4 oz) carton natural low-fat cottage cheese, unlimited green salad items and tomatoes

Mid-afternoon
• 1 fruit choice (see page 18)

Evening
• 1 serving Nutty Chicken*
OR

• 1 average breast of chicken fillet, grilled or baked and skin removed, served with 1 x 175 g (6 oz) baked potato and 4 tablespoons (60 g, 2¹/₂ oz) baked beans

——RECIPE——

Nutty Chicken

Serves 2 at approximately 350 calories per portion

• 225 g (8 oz) chicken fillet without skin
• 50 g (2 oz) natural low-fat yogurt
• 1 tablespoon fresh lime or lemon juice
• Dash chilli sauce or pinch chilli powder
• Little salt and pepper
• 15 g (¹/₂ oz) very low-fat spread
• 110 g (4 oz) broccoli florets
• 110 g (4 oz) mushrooms, sliced
• 1 medium carrot, thinly sliced
• 2 spring onions, chopped
• Little chicken stock
• 4 tablespoons toasted flaked almonds
• 125 g (4¹/₂ oz) boiled rice, preferably brown

Cut the chicken into thin strips. Mix the yogurt with the juice, chilli and seasoning and add to chicken, mixing well. Marinate for an hour if possible.

Heat the very-low-fat spread in a non-stick frying pan and fry the vegetables over a medium heat for a few minutes.

Add the chicken and fry again for a few minutes, stirring all the time. Add a little chicken stock if the mixture sticks at all.

When the chicken is cooked and the vegetables are still firm, add the almonds and rice, stir gently and heat through for 2 minutes, adding a little chicken stock, again, if liked.

TIPS • Most nuts are quite high in calories, but you get 'more for your money' if you use flaked almonds as they weigh very little.

——YOUR ACTIVITIES FOR TODAY——

Body Contouring

Today do one set of standard exercises and one set of super exercises.

Spot Reducing

No spot reducing today.

Fat Burning

Today walk for 40 minutes. Make 30 minutes of your walk brisk.

Aim to cover: 3 miles.

Body Awareness and Tips

Many people with poor body alignment suffer from lower backache. Have you noticed that you are getting fewer aches and pains now? It is because your stomach and back muscles are getting stronger and your back is more supple so you can do more work without putting strain on it.

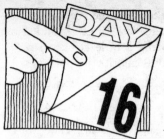

DAILY ALLOWANCES
140 ml (5 fl oz, 1/4 pint)
skimmed milk

UNLIMITEDS
See page 17.

Make full use of your unlimited items during this last week as I have reduced the calories again in your set menus to keep the weight moving off well. Don't forget to drink plenty of water, especially after fat burning exercise.

—— DIET——

Breakfast
• 1 slice wholemeal bread or toast from a large, medium-cut loaf with a very little low-fat spread and 2 teaspoons pure fruit spread
• 1 C-rich fruit choice (see page 18)

Mid-morning
• 1 x 275 ml (10 fl oz, 1/2 pint) glass of mineral water

Lunch
• Egg sandwich: 2 slices wholemeal bread from a large medium-cut loaf with a very little low-fat spread, filled with 1 medium (size 3) hard-boiled egg, sliced, and plenty of sliced cucumber and lettuce

Mid-afternoon
• 1 fruit choice (see page 18)

Evening
• 1 serving Tagliatelle with Mushroom Sauce* with a green side salad; OR
• 110 g (4 oz) extra-lean gammon or sweetcure bacon steak, grilled, served with 140 g (5 oz) instant mashed potato or new potatoes with 75 g (3 oz) peas

——RECIPE——

Tagliatelle with Mushroom Sauce

Serves 2 at approximately 300 calories per portion

• 75 g (3 oz) dried tagliatelle or other pasta of choice,
preferably wholewheat
• 1 dessertspoon corn, olive or sunflower oil
• 110 g (4 oz) lean gammon steak or chicken, cut into strips
• 140 g (5 oz) mushrooms, sliced
• 25 g (1 oz) peas (preferably petit pois)
• 1 teaspoon cornflour
• Vegetable or chicken stock from cube
• 1 x 125 g (4½ oz) tub low-fat natural yogurt
• Salt and pepper to taste
• Fresh chopped parsley

Boil the pasta in plenty of water for the time instructed
on the packet.

While the pasta is cooking, heat oil in a non-stick frying pan and stir-fry the gammon for a few minutes; add
mushrooms and peas and stir for a further minute.

Beat cornflour and a little stock into the yogurt and
add it and the chopped parsley to the pan with seasoning to taste. Cook over gentle heat for a couple of
minutes.

Drain the pasta and serve with sauce.

TIPS • To save sliced bread going stale before you
can eat it all, divide a large loaf into four, bag and
freeze it separately. If you have a microwave it will
take only half a minute or so to defrost. Or you can
toast direct from frozen.

——YOUR ACTIVITIES FOR TODAY——

Body Contouring

Do one set of standard exercises and one set of super exercises.

Spot Reducing

No spot reducing today.

Fat Burning

Walk for 45 minutes. Make 30 of them brisk.
   Aim to cover: 3 miles plus.

Body Awareness and Tips

If you are following the extra body alignment exercise programme, today is the day to do it (see page 201).

Today assess your wardrobe. Decide which clothes really bring out the best in your shape and which don't. It's a fact that however good your shape, some things are never going to look flattering. Clothes that suit you will greatly increase your confidence, so look through the fashion magazines and browse through the shops to discover your own style.

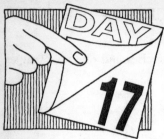

DAILY ALLOWANCES
140 ml (5 fl oz, 1/4 pint)
skimmed milk

UNLIMITEDS
See page 17.

Today it would be a good idea to start reading Chapter 6, all about your maintenance diet, so that you can familiarize yourself with the adaptations you're going to be able to make to your diet and activity programme.

—— DIET——

Breakfast
• 25 g (1 oz) branflakes, Bran Buds or Fruit 'n' Fibre with milk from allowance
• 1 fruit choice (see page 18)

Mid-morning
• 1 Ryvita with a little Marmite (no spread)

Lunch
• 1 x 275 ml (10 oz) can mixed vegetable soup (any variety, but not creamed), and 1 average wholemeal roll; plus 1 satsuma or kiwifruit; OR
• 1 x 100 g (3 1/2 oz) slice of pre-packed vegetable terrine (available from the chilled counter at most super-markets), plus 2 Ryvitas,

served with a large mixed salad; plus 1 C-rich fruit choice (see page 18)

Mid-afternoon
• 1 diet fruit yogurt, any flavour

Evening
• 1 serving Ratatouille Gratin*, with a green salad; OR
• Cheese salad: Grate 40 g (1 1/2 oz) reduced-fat Cheddar-style cheese and mix it with 1 small carrot, grated. Serve tossed in oil-free dressing on a bed of salad greens, plus 1 1/2 slices wholemeal bread from a large medium-cut loaf; plus 1 apple

——RECIPE——

Ratatouille Gratin

• 110 g (4 oz) courgettes
• 225 g (8 oz) aubergine
• 1 tablespoon olive oil
• 1 medium onion, sliced
• 1 clove garlic, crushed (optional)
• 1 medium green pepper, de-seeded and sliced
• 200 g (7 oz) canned, chopped tomatoes
• 1/2 teaspoon ground coriander or chopped basil
• Little salt and pepper
• 1 medium (size 3) egg, beaten
• 140 ml (5 fl oz, 1/4 pint) skimmed milk (extra to allowance)
• 75 g (3 oz) reduced-fat Cheddar-style cheese, grated
• 4 tablespoons fresh breadcrumbs

Slice the courgettes and cut the aubergine into cubes. Sprinkle with salt and leave in a colander to drain for half an hour, to remove any bitterness. Rinse then par-boil in water for a few minutes. Pat dry.

Heat oil in a non-stick pan and stir-fry onion until transparent and just turning golden. Add garlic (if used), aubergine, courgettes and green pepper and stir-fry for a further few minutes.

Add tomatoes and seasoning and simmer, covered, for approximately 30 minutes. Transfer to individual gratin dishes.

Mix together the egg, milk and half the cheese and pour over ratatouille. Sprinkle rest of cheese and bread-crumbs over the top and bake for 25 minutes, until lightly browned and set.

> **TIPS** • For a change, when selecting cheese salad, you could finely chop the apple and add it to the grated cheese and carrot mixture. • You can always parboil aubergines in any recipe that says you should fry them. They soak up tons of fat when fried. Courgettes are less 'greedy', but can still be successfully cooked by parboiling first.

——YOUR ACTIVITIES FOR TODAY——

Body Contouring

Today do one complete standard set and one complete super set. Give it your best!

Spot Reducing

Do your spot reducing programme today at the end of your contouring exercises.

Fat Burning

No fat burning today.

Body Awareness and Tips

If you do a lot of word-processing, typing or computer work, your neck and shoulders are likely to hold a lot of tension. Release the tension every so often by doing the neck and shoulder release exercises in Chapter 5. Check that your chair is supporting your lower back properly so that you don't sit in a 'letter C' position.

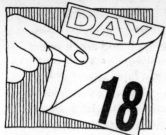

DAILY ALLOWANCES
140 ml (5 fl oz, ¼ pint)
skimmed milk

UNLIMITEDS
See page 17.

On the home straight now. Who says you couldn't stick to a diet programme? You should be feeling really fit and well.

—— DIET——

Breakfast
• 1 x 125 ml (4½ oz) tub French-style set fruit yogurt, any flavour
• 1 C-rich fruit choice (see page 18)

Mid-morning
• 1 x 275 ml (10 fl oz, ½ pint) glass of mineral water

Lunch
• Salmon sandwich: 2 slices of wholemeal bread from a large medium-cut loaf, lightly spread with very-low-fat spread and filled with 50 g (2 oz) pink salmon plus plenty of green salad items

Mid-afternoon
• 1 fruit choice (see page 18)

Evening
• 1 serving Vegetarian Chow Mein* OR
• 175 g (6 oz) white fish fillet, grilled or baked, served with 175 g (6 oz) boiled, baked or instant mashed potato and 110 g (4 oz) broccoli or carrots

TIPS • Chinese dried egg noodles are a boon for busy slimmers. They provide a virtually instant high-carbohydrate, low-fat snack or meal. All you have to do is steep them in a bowl of just boiled water for a few minutes. • For a stronger ginger flavour in the recipe, finely chop the fresh ginger and do not remove it. • Soya sauce is quite salty, but if you buy the 'light' soya sauce the sodium content is much lower and the taste less strong. • Chicken or prawns could be used instead of the tofu, but use a little less as the calorie count is a bit higher.

——RECIPE——

Vegetarian Chow Mein

Serves 2 at approximately 305 calories per portion

• Scant tablespoon corn or sunflower oil
• 110 g (4 oz) smoked tofu, cut into thin strips
• 50 g (2 oz) red pepper, de-seeded and chopped
• 2 spring onions, chopped
• 50 g (2 oz) sweetcorn
• 50 g (2 oz) beansprouts
• 1/2 teaspoon garlic purée (optional)
• 1 small piece fresh ginger or 1/2 teaspoon dried
• 1 dessertspoon soya sauce
• 1 dessertspoon dry sherry
• 1 teaspoon cornflour
• Little water
• 75 g (3 oz) medium egg noodles, cooked as instructed on packet

Heat the oil in a non-stick frying pan and stir-fry the tofu strips until golden. Remove with a slatted spoon.

Stir-fry the red pepper, onions, sweetcorn and beansprouts for a few minutes with the garlic (if used) and ginger.

Mix together the soya sauce, sherry, cornflour and water, add to pan with the tofu and stir-fry for a minute.

Add the noodles and stir to heat through. If you have used fresh ginger, remove it before serving.

——YOUR ACTIVITIES FOR TODAY——

Body Contouring
No body contouring today.

Spot Reducing
Do your spot reducing routine at the end of your fat-burning programme.

Fat Burning
Today walk for 45 minutes. Cover the middle 30 minutes at a brisk pace.

Aim to cover: 3 miles plus.

Body Awareness and Tips
I hope you've gained some useful information from the instant slimming and body awareness techniques. Don't give up on what you've begun to practise once the 21 days are over – they are habits that will help to keep your body looking great throughout the rest of your life – and the correct alignment will help you to better health, too.

Today, do the 10-minute body re-alignment programme on page 201.

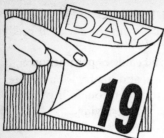

DAILY ALLOWANCES
140 ml (5 fl oz, 1/4 pint)
skimmed milk

UNLIMITEDS
See page 17.

Only three days to go, so be careful to control portion sizes for the last days. It's always worth weighing the higher-calorie items such as cheese and potatoes so that you don't cheat accidentally.

—— DIET——

Breakfast
• 1 slice wholemeal bread or toast from a large, medium-cut loaf with a very little low-fat spread and 2 teaspoons pure fruit spread
• 1 C-rich fruit choice (see page 18)

Mid-morning
• 1 x 275 ml (10 fl oz, 1/2 pint) glass of mineral water

Lunch
• 25 g (1 oz) Brie, Camembert or Edam cheese, or 75 g (3 oz) cottage cheese; plus 3 Ryvitas, dark rye or oatbran, and a large mixed salad; plus 1 medium banana; OR

• Sandwich of 2 slices wholemeal bread from large medium-cut loaf with a little very low-fat spread, filled with 50 g (2 oz) half-fat cream cheese, e.g., Philadelphia Light, unlimited green salad items and sliced tomatoes

Mid-afternoon
• 1 fruit choice (see page 18)

Evening
• 1 serving Curried Chicken Baked Potatoes* with a green salad; OR
• 1 x 225 g (8 oz) jacket potato served with 140 g (5 oz) baked beans

——RECIPE——

Curried Chicken Baked Potatoes

Serves 2 at approximately 300 calories per portion

- 2 x 200 g (7 oz) baking potatoes
- 3 tablespoons natural low-fat yogurt
- 1 level teaspoon mild curry powder or tikka paste
- 1 teaspoon lemon juice
- Salt and pepper to taste
- 110 g (4 oz) cooked chicken meat (no skin), cut into small pieces
- 25 g (1 oz) no-need-to-soak apricot halves, chopped
- 50 g (2 oz) green or red pepper, de-seeded and chopped small

Scrub and prick the potatoes, and bake them at 200°C (400°F) for an hour or until soft.

Cut tops off, scoop out flesh and mash with a little of the yogurt and seasoning.

Meanwhile, mix rest of yogurt with curry powder, lemon juice and seasoning and toss it with the chicken, apricots and green and red pepper.

Put mashed potato back into shells and heat through for a few minutes if necessary. Top with chicken mixture and serve.

TIPS • In summer, you could substitute 200 g (7 oz) diced cold boiled new potatoes for the baked potato and turn the recipe dish into a curred chicken and potato salad. • Remember not to eat your evening meal too late at night. Between 6 and 7 p.m. is ideal. If this is not always possible, try to leave at least 2 hours before eating and going to bed.

——YOUR ACTIVITIES FOR TODAY——

Body Contouring
Do two super sets today. Keep up the pace, and really work your body.

Spot Reducing
No spot reducing today.

Fat Burning
Today walk 45 minutes. Make 35 of them brisk.
  Aim to cover: 3½ miles.
  If you're doing an aerobic alternative instead of the walking programme, you should be doing your chosen alternative (or combination of them) for at least 20 minutes per session by now.

Body Awareness and Tips
Do you always go to sleep in the same position? This can easily create body misalignment over the years. Try to vary between lying facing one side and the other and sometimes lie on your back. A firmish mattress and not having your pillows too high will also help you to maintain a good sleeping position. Sleep with the window open to create an oxygen-rich environment.

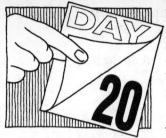

DAILY ALLOWANCES
140 ml (5 fl oz, ¹/₄ pint)
skimmed milk

UNLIMITEDS
See page 17.

As you will by now have some clothes that are no longer fitting you very well, see if there is anything you can re-vamp. For instance, a now-baggy shift dress might be shortened and turned into a big over-leggings top. Or a favourite skirt could be taken in. It's worth investing in some new bras and briefs, though, or lycra-fit bodysuits for colder weather. They give your body an even better outline.

—— DIET ——

Breakfast
• 25 g (1 oz) branflakes, bran buds or fruit 'n' fibre with milk from allowance
• 1 C-rich fruit choice (see page 18)

Mid-morning
• 1 x 275 ml (10 fl oz, ¹/₂ pint) glass of mineral water

Lunch
1 x 225 g (8 oz) can of baked beans in tomato sauce on 1 slice wholemeal toast from a large, medium-cut loaf; OR

• Sandwich of 2 slices wholemeal bread from a large medium-cut loaf filled with 50 g (2 oz) extra-lean roast beef, 1 teaspoon horseradish sauce and unlimited green salad items

Mid-afternoon
• 1 fruit choice (see page 18)

Evening
• 1 serving Herby Prawns with Courgettes* with 4 tablespoons boiled rice and a green salad; OR
• 75 g (3 oz) peeled prawns

with a large mixed salad, plus 1 average wholemeal roll and 1 teaspoon reduced- calorie mayonnaise; plus 1 fruit choice (see page 18)

——RECIPE——

Herby Prawns with Courgettes
Serves 2 at approximately 230 calories per portion

- 325 g (12 oz) courgettes
- 1 dessertspoon corn, olive or sunflower oil
- 1 small onion, finely chopped
- 1/2 teaspoon garlic purée (optional)
- 1 teaspoon Mediterranean mixed herbs
- 1 tablespoon tomato purée
- 200 g (7 oz) chopped, canned tomatoes
- 225 g (8 oz) peeled prawns
- Salt and black pepper to taste

Slice the courgettes into thin rounds, put them in a colander, sprinkle with salt and leave to drain for half an hour. Rinse and pat dry.

Heat the oil in a non-stick frying pan and stir-fry the onion until it is transparent and just turning golden.

Add garlic purée and courgettes and stir-fry for several minutes until courgettes are turning golden.

Add herbs, tomato purée and tomatoes and simmer, covered, for 15–20 minutes.

Add prawns and cook for a further 2 minutes. Check the taste – you may want to add a little salt or salt substitute before serving.

> **TIPS** • Cook some extra rice for your lunchtime salad tomorrow. Plain boiled rice is much more interesting, and nicer to look at, if you add either a teaspoon of turmeric powder to the boiling water to give it a yellow colour, or a very little wild rice, which is black. Remember, however, that wild rice needs to be cooked for up to 45 minutes. You could cook some in a batch and freeze it in little containers. Simply defrost and add to your long-grain rice for the last few cooking minutes. The usual proportion of wild rice to plain rice is 1:8.

——YOUR ACTIVITIES FOR TODAY——

Body Contouring
No body contouring today.

Spot Reducing
Do your spot reducing routine today after the fat burning programme.

Fat Burning
Walk for 45 minutes. Make 35 of them brisk.
  Aim to cover: $3^1/2$ miles plus.

Body Awareness and Tips
Do your 10-minute body re-alignment programme today (see page 201).
  Read Chapter 5 through again and check that you are still maintaining all your correct alignments.

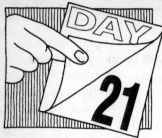

DAILY ALLOWANCES
140 ml (5 fl oz, 1/2 pint)
skimmed milk

UNLIMITEDS
See page 17.

It's your last day, so enjoy it and look forward to weighing and measuring yourself tomorrow morning.

—— DIET——

Breakfast
• 1 slice wholemeal bread or toast from a large medium-cut loaf with a little very-low-fat spread and 2 teaspoons pure fruit spread
• 1 C-rich fruit choice (see page 18)

Mid-morning
• 1 x 275 ml (10 fl oz, 1/2 pint) glass of mineral water

Lunch
• Rice Salad: Mix 140 g (5 oz) cooked cool rice with 50 g (2 oz) peeled prawns or tuna, 50 g (2 oz) green pepper, de-seeded and chopped, and 50 g (2 oz) chopped pineapple. Toss all in an oil-free French dressing and serve on a bed of green salad; OR

• Tuna sandwich: Fill 2 slices wholemeal bread from a large medium-cut loaf with 1 x 100 g (3 1/2 oz) can of tuna in brine, drained, and cucumber, cress and lettuce.

Mid-afternoon
• 1 fruit choice (see page 18)

Evening
• 1 serving Soufflé Omelette* with 1 slice wholemeal bread from a large medium-cut loaf and a green salad; OR
• 1 medium (size 3) egg, poached, served on 1 slice wholemeal bread from a large medium-cut loaf; plus 1 fruit choice and 1 large banana

——RECIPE——

Soufflé Omelette

Serves 2 at approximately 230 calories per portion

- 50 g (2 oz) button mushrooms, sliced
- 50 g (2 oz) beansprouts
- 1 teaspoon soya sauce
- 4 small (size 4) eggs, separated
- 15 g (½ oz) butter
- Pinch dry mustard
- Salt and pepper to taste

Mix mushrooms, raw beansprouts and soya sauce together.

In a clean bowl, whisk the egg whites until they form peaks that hold their shape.

Whisk yolks, mustard and seasoning to taste, then fold yolk mixture into whites.

Heat half the butter in a small omelette pan until foaming. Add half the egg mixture and cook until bottom is golden.

Place half of the mushroom mixture on one half of the omelette, slide out on to a plate and fold over. Make the second omelette in same way.

TIPS • Making an omelette is probably the one occasion when you really do need to use butter in the cooking pan, rather than oil or low-fat spread. It is the only type of fat I've found that gives that really golden colour to your omelette – and that extra special taste! But you could, of course, use 2 teaspoons of corn oil instead, if you prefer.

——YOUR ACTIVITIES FOR TODAY——

Body Contouring

Do two sets of super exercises today.

Spot Reducing

Do your spot reducing routine at the end of your contouring.

Fat Burning

Walk for 45 minutes. Make 35 of those minutes brisk.
   Aim to cover: 3 1/2 miles plus.

Body Awareness and Tips

It's weigh and measure time in the morning, so get an early night and sleep well after three weeks of really good healthy body work!

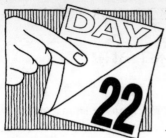

NEXT MORNING

TODAY I WEIGH
_____ stone_____ lbs (_____ kg)

TODAY I MEASURE
Bust:_____ Waist:_____ Stomach:_____ Hips:_____

I HAVE LOST A TOTAL OF
_____ lbs (_____ kg)

I HAVE LOST A TOTAL OF
_____ ins (_____ cm)

MY DRESS SIZE HAS GONE DOWN FROM

A SIZE_____ TO A SIZE_____

WELL DONE!

Now turn to the maintenance programme in Chapter 6 or, if you wish to repeat the programme, see the note on page 23 before you start.

Chapter 2
BODY CONTOURING

Your dress size depends as much on the shape you're in as it does on the weight you are. And that is why, during your 21-day programme, the exercise and activity you do is just as important as what and how much you eat.

And that is why it is vital that you do the body contouring programme five days a week during the 21 days. The system is simple, yet it is incredibly effective.

Body contouring is a unique form of exercise. It is not just a conditioning routine (though it will certainly do that); not even just a toning routine. It can actually re-shape you in the best way for your individual body, slimming you down, firming you up and adding shape where you need it.

Body contouring, combined with the spot reducing, fat burning and body awareness sections of the programme, will help you to lose that dress size (or sizes) by whittling away inches where they need to go. But it won't leave you thin or shapeless – you'll have the feminine, yet firm, shape that is so right for the '90s.

Just in case you think, 'Ah well, she's not thinking of me! I could never do that, why not strip off to your pants and get your husband, mum or best friend to take a full-length photo of you as you are now? Get them to take another in three weeks' time and I guarantee if you do the body contouring and complementary routines properly and diligently for the next three weeks, the difference will amaze you.

Before You Begin

But before you start the routine it is very, very important that you first read all the notes that follow. These notes are to help you benefit the most from your programme; they are also for your own safety.

Best Time of Day

What time of day should you do your body contouring routine? As a general rule, on the days when you have no fat burning programme to do (see individual days of the programme) it is of no great consequence what time of day you do the routine. However, most people best perform this type of exercise when they leave at least an hour after a meal, but don't leave it till late in the evening as you are likely to be too tired to perform well. If you go to work, therefore, I suggest you do the exercises when you get up or soon after you get home in the evening.

On the days when you do body contouring and fat burning (see individual days' instructions on the programme in Chapter 1), the ideal is to have a few hours' gap between the two. Do body contouring in the morning and fat burning in the early evening, or vice versa. If that isn't possible, then do your body contouring directly after your fat burning.

Clothing

You must wear an outfit that allows full range of movement. Never try to exercise in jeans or anything that cuts into your stomach, such as a tight waistband or a leather belt. Very baggy clothes are also not ideal as they may hinder movement, and stop you from seeing exactly what your body is doing – an important part of exercising correctly.

So if you don't have a leotard or other exercise wear, perhaps the next best thing is a pair of leggings, or a pair of shorts with an elasticated waistband, and a sleeveless T-shirt or vest.

There is no need to wear a bra with a leotard, but if you are wearing a bra it should be one with elasticated straps that won't keep falling off your shoulders when you move. Stopping to hoist straps back up every few minutes is a distraction you can do without.

For the body contouring routine there is no need to wear training shoes, as it involves no jarring leg work. You can go barefoot, if you like, but socks and jazz shoes are ideal; they are very flexible and perfect for floor work. You can, of course, wear trainers, if you prefer; the lighter and more flexible they are, the better. I wouldn't wear training boots as they restrict your ankle movement too much.

Lastly, if the room in which you plan to exercise is warm you should have no need to wear extra clothing for the warm-up. But, if for any reason you don't feel perfectly warm as you are about to start your body contouring routine, do the warm-up in a tracksuit or jumper, and legwarmers – anything non-restrictive to keep your muscles from strain – until you are warm, at which point you should remove the extra clothes.

The Room

Decide where you are going to do your exercises. For the body contouring and spot reducing programmes, you simply need a space long enough to lie full length with your arms stretched out – and wide enough so that you can stretch out to the left and to the right without fear of hitting anything! Also consider overhead lights and make sure you're not going to smash them and yourself when doing arm reaches!

Ideally, your exercise room should have a nice thick carpet and be floorboarded, rather than an unyielding surface, such as concrete. If your room isn't carpeted, I advise you to invest in a cushioned exercise mat (available from sports shops or by mail order) as you won't find exercising on stripped pine or parquet very kind to your bones. I would never advise you to use a towel over polished wood flooring; it is far too easy to slip. If your floor isn't carpeted, wear exercise shoes and socks.

Lastly, your room should be warm enough. If you exercise in the cold, your muscles will start off cold and that's bad for two reasons. First, they don't perform as well as warm muscles, therefore you will find the routine harder to do. And, secondly, cold muscles risk strain, tearing and injury much more than warm muscles. Imagine your muscles are like a piece of plasticine. When it's cold it's hard to mould into shape, and if you pull it, it snaps. When plasticine is warm it's easy to 'work', and when pulled it just stretches easily. Muscles have the added advantage of contracting back into shape after they've been stretched if they are exercised sensibly and not over-strained ... something plasticine can't do.

I can't stress enough the importance of having warm, pliable muscles for the body contouring and spot reducing exercises, so if for any reason at the end of the warm-up you don't feel really warm, do it again, find more heat, or whatever. But don't start the routine.

Extras

To start with, you may find a small cushion is helpful for the stomach exercises. You may also like to spread a towel out on your carpet both to save your carpet and to save you getting carpet fibres in your lungs when lying on your tummy. Remember: don't lay a towel on polished wooden floors (see above).

If you want to, you can do the exercises to music, as long as the beat of music doesn't force you to do the exercises too quickly. Your exercises should be rhythmic, but they should also be controlled. If the music helps your rhythm, fine, but if it makes you lose control, then it's wrong. Music that you find appropriate when you begin the routine will not be appropriate after a few days, for you will be doing the exercises slightly faster.

——THE ROUTINE——

I expect you're impatient to start exercising, but please stay with me a few minutes longer. I'm going to take you through the complete contouring programme because it's vital that you know what you're doing and why you're doing it, to get the most out of any routine.

The contouring programme consists of a warm-up, a set of 12 core exercises and, finally, a cool-down.

The Warm-Up
The warm-up consists of seven simple movements and should take you approximately 3 minutes to complete. The warm-up is an essential part of the routine because it releases your joints, banishes stiffness and literally warms up the major muscles. Put some effort into the warm-up, it isn't a waste of your time.

The 12 Core Exercises
Do these 12 exercises in the correct sequence. Each exercise has a standard version. This is the version that you should start with.

The 12 exercises are movements repeated in sets of 10. You begin by doing one set of each exercise (or part of a set, if you find one complete set too difficult at first).

It is very, very important to read the instructions accompanying each exercise before you begin, and to be certain that you understand what you're reading. Practise the positions and movements for each exercise before you begin a real routine. The correct technique for any exercise in the programme is more important than other factors, such as the number of repetitions. For instance, if you position your body wrongly, you may well be exercising the wrong part of your body. That's why it's much better to manage half a set well, than to do two sets incorrectly.

It is important to concentrate on the area of your body that you're working, and to relax, as far as possible, the rest of your body. Breathe normally throughout, unless instructed otherwise. It is also vital to be in control of the exercise. No wild movements, no flinging or jerking of arms and legs. Pace is an important factor. For the first few days maintain a slow to steady rhythm. Later, try for a steady rhythm and when you are proficient you can keep up a steady to fast rhythm. If you try to do the exercises too quickly before you are ready, you will lose control and concentration. Then it's more likely that you'll carry out the exercises incorrectly and get little or no benefit from them.

Remember! It's not just what you do, but how you do it that's important to the success of this routine.

Now a word about your ability. Everyone's body is different. Some of the exercises you will naturally find easier, and some harder. As a guide, you are achieving the correct response to an exercise if at the end of one set you feel you have worked the body area in question.

You are underworking if you feel no effort at all, and you are overworking if you feel pain, severe muscle tremble or, with the stomach exercises, muscle bulge.

Never push your body if you feel actual pain. Stop the exercise at once. The body contouring exercises are based on generally recognized safety standards and shouldn't cause pain if you follow the guidelines. On the other hand, if you don't put effort into your routine, you won't improve, and your body shape won't improve. Effort is crucial. And determination and commitment are equally important.

For instance, if you find one particular exercise more difficult than the others, your inclination may be to skip that exercise. That is exactly what you shouldn't be doing. If an exercise is hard for you, that means that the part of the body it is supposed to be working is particularly out of shape and is in need of more work on it, not less. Let's give you an example. You may find that on Exercise 6, the Hip Lift, you're getting virtually no movement. This means that your lower abdominal muscles are particularly weak and need extra work. Keep at that particular exercise with more determination. Don't give up!

Progressing

So once you have mastered the basic 12-exercise routine, how do you progress? Without progression, you can't improve. You do this in three ways:

• You continue to perform the exercises better. For instance, on Exercise 2, the Shoulder Pulls, you will concentrate on raising your upper body further off the floor in each movement. Guidelines on how to improve your performance of each exercise appear in the text accompanying the photographs.

• You increase the number of repeats that you do. When you have mastered one set of 10 and can do it easily, try two sets with a short rest in between. It is also useful in between sets to perform a stretch to ease the muscle that has been working. Guidance on suitable stretches appears, again, in the photo text.

Doing two or more sets will not necessarily mean that the contouring programme will take you much longer to complete. By the time you are ready for more sets you will be performing the exercises at maximum advisable pace; in other words, you're working much harder in the same timespan.

• You move on to the super version of each exercise. The super version is simply a harder variation of the standard exercise, and should not be attempted until the standard version has been completely mastered. And when beginning the super exercises you should do just one set at first.

IMPORTANT NOTE: For more guidance on progress, read the notes under Your Activities for Today for each day of the 21-day programme in Chapter 1. The notes there suggest when to increase sets and when to move on to the super exercises. These suggestions are for guidance only. If you are not ready to progress as suggested, don't feel that you've 'failed'. Simply delay progressing until you are ready.

The Cool-Down

The cool-down consists of seven stretching exercises and should take approximately 2–3 minutes. Stretches are very important at the end of any exercise routine. You can really feel your muscles thanking you for stretching them out at the end of a period of hard work! Tension is created in the muscles when they work, and stretching removes that tension, ensuring that you won't wake up the following day feeling achey and sore. Stretching also helps you to achieve a streamlined shape to your muscles rather than 'bulk', and it elongates the waist and helps posture, too. (For more on posture and stretching, read Chapter 5.)

For stretches to work properly, they need to be held for a minimum of 10 seconds, at the exact point when you feel the stretch really working – not discomfort, not pain, but the muscle telling you, 'That's it – I don't want to go any further than that today.' It helps very much if you relax into your stretches. If you feel yourself tensing up, take a big breath, relax and you'll find you can stretch that bit further.

The stretches that cause most people the most problem are the Groin and Hamstring Stretches (Stretches 6 and 7). Don't worry, just enjoy the stretches and you will see yourself getting more supple every day. Never attempt stretches when you aren't warmed up.

Now we are ready to begin running through the routine. Don't forget to acclimatize yourself to the exercises first, before you attempt a whole routine in 20 minutes. Also, for maximum benefit, don't forget to use the body contouring programme in conjunction with the notes for each day in the 21-day programme.

Don't forget, before starting this or any other exercise routine, it is advisable to check with your doctor that the exercise programme is suitable for you.

——BODY CONTOURING—— THE WARM-UP

Warm-up 1: Shoulder Rolls

Stand with legs hip-width apart, arms relaxed at sides, tummy and bottom tucked in (see note below on the pelvic tilt). Get upper back as straight as possible without tensing, and neck as long as possible. Now make a circle with your right shoulder. Bring it forward, then up, then back and down to start. The movement should flow. Do 15 circles, relax arm and repeat with left shoulder.

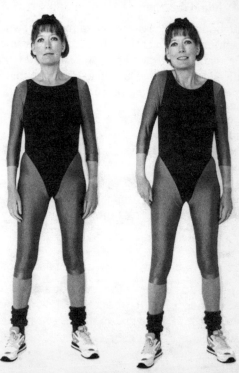

Tips

Keep chin down. Prevent it from coming up, as this will create tension in the back of your neck. As the shoulder comes round to the back, try to feel the shoulder blade working.

Improving

When you've accomplished the single shoulder rolls, you can do both shoulders together. If one shoulder is stiffer than the other, do extra rolls on that side.

The Pelvic Tilt

Throughout this exercise programme the pelvic tilt will be mentioned frequently. This is a simple movement which assures that the pelvis, stomach and lower back are aligned correctly. The pelvic tilt is the main key to better looks and better posture. When doing all the

Pelvic Tilt (lying)

WRONG

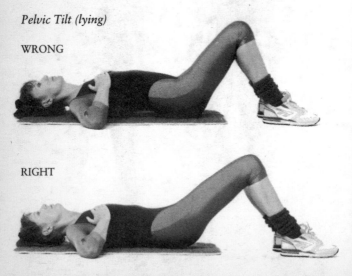

RIGHT

exercises, your pelvis should not tip forward (a position many of us adopt all the time and which causes the tummy to 'tip' outwards), but should sit like a cup. Your tummy tucks in, your bottom tucks under and any exaggerated curve in your lower back is eliminated. For more information on posture and the importance of the correct pelvic tilt, turn to Chapter 5.

Exercises should never be carried out without ensuring the pelvis is in this correct alignment.

Pelvic Tilt (standing)

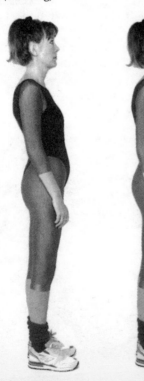

WRONG   RIGHT

Warm-Up 2: Arm Circles/Knee Bends

Now your shoulders are warm you can proceed to large arm circles, coupled with knee bends, to warm up some larger muscles and get the heart going, too.

Stand with legs wide apart, as shown, feet pointing outwards to 45 degrees. Now, keeping your tummy in and, your back as upright as possible, bend your knees and at the same time, sweep your arms across you and out to the sides in a big, circling motion. Rise up as the circle ends.

Bend your knees again, and this time sweep both arms back in a large circle, feeling your shoulders and back muscles work.

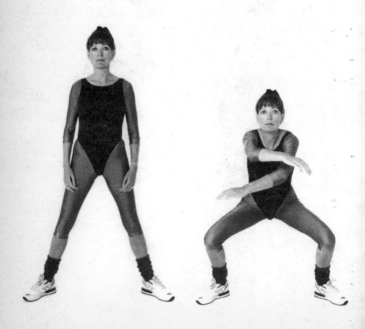

Do 20 knee bends coupled with 10 cross body arm circles and 10 backward arm circles.

Tips

There's no need to bend really low – you should never dip below knee level in any case. Make sure your feet are far enough apart to make the exercise comfortable.

Concentrate on getting your arm circles wide and on breathing steadily. Don't hold your breath!

Improving

Your backward arm circles will become bigger (you'll be able to get them further back) and you will be able to dip without leaning forwards. Concentrate on keeping that tummy pulled in as you go.

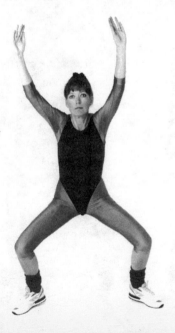

Warm-Up 3: Hip Circling

You need to mobilize the hip joints and warm up your tummy now. Stand with your legs slightly more than hip-width apart, knees slightly bent, arms relaxed. Now circle your hips clockwise while keeping the rest of your body as still as possible. Do 10 circles, stop, then repeat 10 anti-clockwise.

Tips

In order to keep the rest of your body still, you'll really have to use your tummy and bottom to work those hips round. Concentrate on feeling them working as you go.

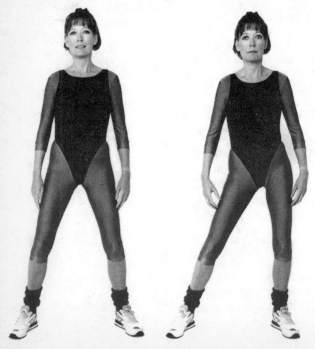

Improving

Do bigger and bigger circles, eventually aiming to keep your knees and chest completely still.

Warm-Up 4: Lower Back Release

Stand with your feet hip-width apart, hands resting lightly on thighs and with upper body slightly forward and relaxed, knees slightly bent. Now do an exaggerated Pelvic Tilt, bringing bottom under, pulling stomach in and rounding out your lower back, all in one strong movement. As you do so, your knees will bend more and your upper body will move forward into a curve.

Relax and repeat the move 10 times.

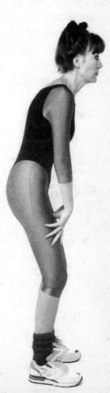

Tips

If you're doing this correctly, your stomach will 'disappear' in towards your back. The movement should be strong but not jerky.

Improving

Really get that back rounding out and the stomach will concave in. Practise breathing in as you relax, and out as you do the move.

107

Warm-Up 5: Reach and Lift

Warm up your sides, back and calves all in one movement, which also helps balance and coordination. Stand
with legs hip-width apart, knees soft, not locked. Do a
Pelvic Tilt – pulling tummy in and
bottom under – and maintain the
correct tilt throughout. Now raise
your right arm up towards the
ceiling, feeling a stretch all along
your right side, and at the same
time rise up on to the balls of
your feet. As you bring the arm
down, bring your feet down, too.
Now reach for the ceiling with
your left arm, rising up again.

Do 20 reach and lifts, 10 on
each side, alternately.

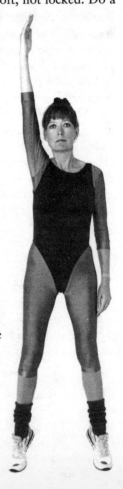

Tips

If you find the movement hard at
first, do the arm reaches followed
by the heel lifts. Don't raise your
eyes to the ceiling, just look
straight ahead. You want to keep
your neck still and concentrate the
work in your sides and back. Be
careful not to tip forwards as you
rise.

Improving

Aim to reach higher; try to lift
your heels higher. Hold each
reach and lift a little longer.

Warm-Up 6: Waist Twists

Warm up the waist area with gentle twists. Stand, feet hip-width apart, fingers on shoulders and elbows up. Now, keeping your hips as still as possible and facing square to the front, twist your body from waist upwards round to the right, moving your head round, too, to look over your shoulder. Return to start and twist to other side.

Do 10 twists to each side.

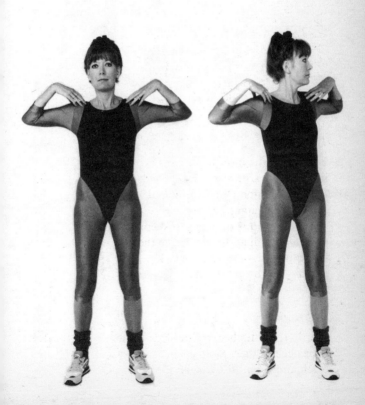

Tips

Do the twists in a slow and controlled manner. It's more important to keep your hips square to the front than it is to be able to twist round a long way.

Improving

As the days go by, you will be able to twist further, thus whittling your waist away a little as you warm up!

Warm-Up 7: Knee Lifts

Lastly, you want to loosen up your bottom, outer thighs and hips and get the heart pumping to ensure you go

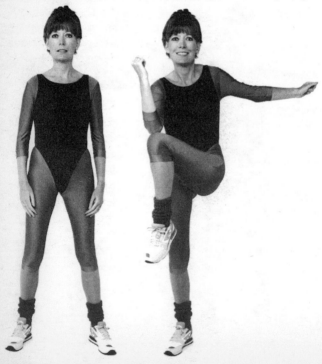

into your core routine warmed up in every respect.

Stand with your feet apart and with much of your weight over the right foot. Maintaining the Pelvic Tilt, bring your left knee up and across your body, bring your right elbow down towards your left knee and raise your left arm up and out to the side.

Do 10 knee lifts on this side, then transfer the weight to your left leg and repeat 10 times with the right knee.

Tips

The sequence should be fun and energetic, like dancing. Really put some effort into the movement; feel light on

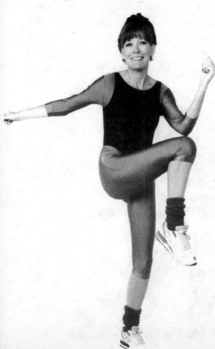

your 'lifting' foot so that it hardly touches the floor when it returns.

Improving

Keep your back as straight as possible throughout, and concentrate on getting your right arm out wide as your left foot returns to the floor.

——BODY CONTOURING——
THE EXERCISES

Exercise 1: Press-Ups

Standard

Press-ups are brilliant for contouring the whole of your upper body and upper arms. By utilizing muscles you didn't know existed, they re-shape your 'pecs' (the muscles that give your bust a nice shape), and totally eliminate that horrid 'loose flesh' women often get at the backs of their arms as they get older.

For the standard version, kneel square on all fours with your arms slightly wider apart than body width and with your fingers pointing in a little. Do the Pelvic Tilt so that your tummy disappears into your body and your lower back flattens. Keep your neck in line with

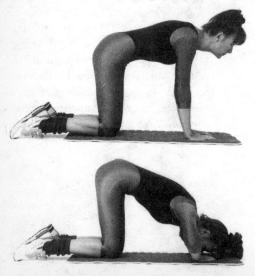

your back. Now bend your elbows and, still keeping your back flat and rigid, dip your head down to the floor, then raise up again. One set equals 10 of these press-ups.

When you've finished, shake your arms out for a few seconds. If doing more sets, do the Triceps Stretch between sets (see page 137).

Tips

If your arms start to shake at any stage during your first set, or after – Stop. This exercise is harder than it looks. But don't give up – you will improve rapidly if you do the exercise regularly. You may find you can complete a set if you have a rest halfway through.

Improving

Make sure your head touches the floor each time you dip. Move your knees a little further back for a slightly harder version.

Super

Start with your legs much further back as shown. Lift your lower legs and cross your ankles. Now do the press-ups as before, in sets of 10. Remember, only move on to the super version when you have completely mastered the standard version.

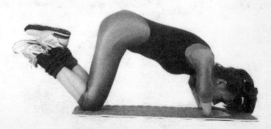

Exercise 2: The Ship

Standard

This exercise position and movement reminds me of a ship sailing through waves. It is the best at contouring your middle and upper back and at strengthening your shoulders. It also gives your chest a fine stretch. Anyone who works at a desk all day will find this difficult at first!

Lie on your tummy and clasp your hands behind your back as shown. Keeping your legs still, lift your head, neck and chest off the floor, at the same time moving your hands down towards your legs. Relax and repeat 10 times for one set.

Tips

If you have very weak shoulders and a tight chest you may find it nearly impossible to get more than an inch (2.5 cm) off the floor at first. Concentrate on squeezing the shoulder blades together and on pulling your hands down across your bottom. Breathe out as you come up; in as you relax. Do a Back Stretch (see page 136) between sets.

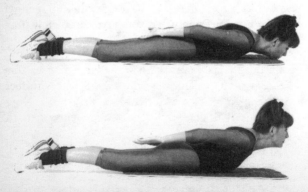

Improving

The further up you can come, the stronger you are getting and the more deeply you are re-shaping yourself. Stop yourself from pressing your hipbones into the floor to get extra lift. Hips and legs should be relaxed.

Super

Come up as in the standard version, but this time continue the movement by bringing the arms out to your sides and round to rest on the floor in front of you. Then relax. This is a motion very much like the butterfly swimming stroke.

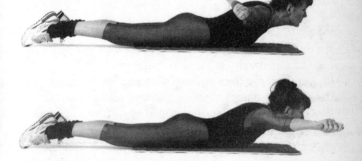

Exercise 3: Arm Pumps

Standard

The third and last 'pecs' and shoulder exercise, this sequence uses the weight of your arms. Stand with feet hip-width apart and knees soft. Do the Pelvic Tilt. Now you're going to do three different arm movements, each in sets of 10.

First, raise arms out in front of you at shoulder level, hands forming fists. Now pull your arms out to the sides

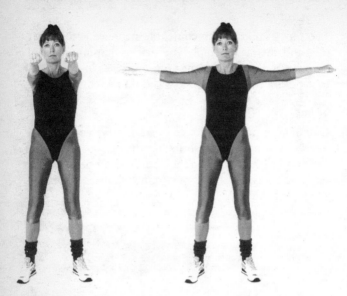

making sure arms remain parallel to floor. Return to start and repeat.

Second, start with arms at sides. Now lift them up and out and up to touch above your head, making two wide straight semi-circles as you go. Bring them back down as wide as you can and repeat.

Third, start with your arms up and out to the sides, elbows bent so arms form two L-shapes and shoulder blades are squeezed together. Now bring elbows round to the front so that lower arms meet in front of your chest. Really squeeze, then pull back out again and repeat. Do a Triceps Stretch (see page 137) between sets.

Tips

Concentrate all the while on feeling your pecs and shoulders work. Your shoulders must be down throughout,

116

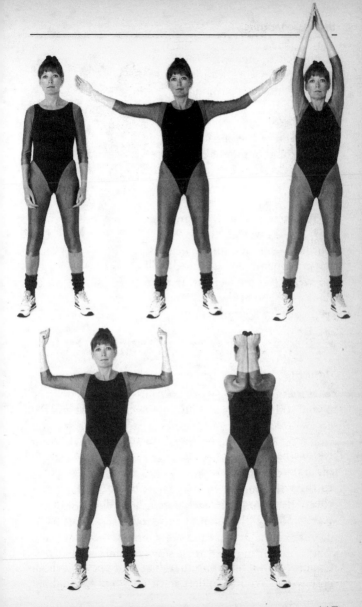

117

not hunched, otherwise you'll develop the wrong outline and you'll create neck tension.

Improving

Watch you're keeping your tummy tight throughout and aim to put much more effort into each move.

Super

All the same routine but now add 3 lb (1.5 kg) weights to the routine. If you don't have weights, two cooking oil bottles (filled) will do. When picking weights up from the floor, bend at the knee and keep your back straight.

Exercise 4: Curl-Ups

Standard

Now we're beginning work on your stomach. You need to work on your upper stomach, lower stomach and the muscles that cross from your ribcage to your waist if you want a really firm stomach and slim waist. This curl-up concentrates on the upper stomach but the lower stomach will get some work, too.

Lie on the floor with your knees bent. Do the Pelvic Tilt so that your lower back flattens into the floor. Place your hands lightly behind your ears as shown. Breathing out, raise your head and shoulders off the floor using your stomach muscles, then slowly come back to the floor, breathing in as you do so. 10 repeats equals one set. Do a Stomach Stretch (see page 135) between sets.

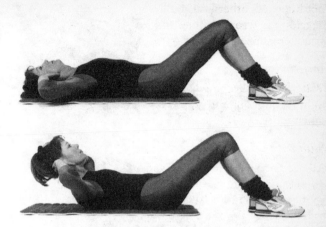

Tips

To ensure that your stomach does the work and not your neck, make sure that you keep approximately a 3-inch (7.5 cm) distance between your chin and chest. While you curl up, look up to the ceiling rather than towards your knees. Your shoulders and neck should come off the floor at the same time. Never drag your neck. Don't use your hands to pull up your head.

Improving

Rise further off the floor, but there is no need to come all the way up. Your stomach works hardest for the first 45 degrees.

Super

The super version of curl-ups works the lower abdomen equally hard. Lie on your back with lower back flat as before. Now bring your knees in towards your chest, let your thighs fall open and cross your feet. With hands

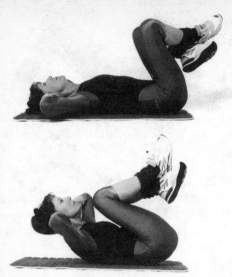

placed as before, curl up, but this time lift your bottom off the floor, bringing your knees in a little further as you do so.

Relax and repeat 10 times for one set.

Exercise 5: Rotated Curl-Ups I

Standard

These exercises predominantly work the obliques (the sides of the stomach), muscles that are normally severely underused. The good news is that they are quick to respond to the right work, giving you a waist to be proud of.

Start in the standard curl-ups position. Resting your right elbow on the floor, bring your left shoulder up and over so that your left elbow heads towards your right knee. Breathe out as you come up.

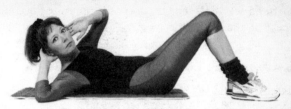

Slowly return to the floor and repeat 10 times on that side. Rest your left elbow on the floor and repeat to your right side.

Tips

Don't bring your moving elbow in to create the impression of coming up further – your rising arms should stay in the same position. It is the shoulder that moves.

Improving

Concentrate on coming up and over your body in a rounded movement. As you get stronger you will be able to reach further and further across.

Super

This brings in the lower tummy area, too. Lie in the starting position for curl-ups. Now cross your right leg over your left knee as shown. Each time you do a rotated curl-up, bring the legs in so that the rotated elbow meets the opposite knee (or as near as you can get).

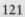

121

After a set of 10 repeats, cross the opposite knee and repeat on the other side.

Exercise 6: Hip Lifts

Standard

The hip lift is the best exercise for flattening out the stomach area below the 'belly button', a notoriously difficult area to work. Lie on your back with knees bent and lower back flattened to the floor, arms resting across your chest as shown. Now bring your knees in above your stomach and cross your feet. Using a small but rhythmic motion, try to lift your bottom and hips off the floor and straight up into the air.

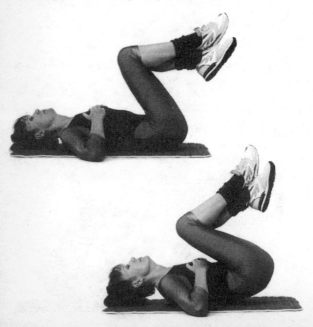

Tips

Don't rock violently in an attempt to lever yourself up.
Concentrate on using the stomach to pull up your bottom.

Don't use your hands to push yourself off the floor.

Improving

Place your fingers over your lower abdomen and feel the
muscles working as you lift. Concentrate on targeting all
movement into the hips and bottom.

Super

Lie in the same starting position but this time bring your
legs in and then up until not quite straight. Now per-

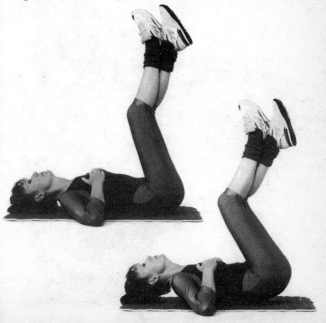

form a very small movement, trying to push your feet up further towards the ceiling by using your lower stomach. The feet shouldn't rock towards your head; they should only move upwards.

One set is 10 lifting movements. If doing more sets, hold knees in to your chest to relax.

Exercise 7: Side Leg Raises

Standard

Now we move on to hip and thigh exercises. People who spend much of the day sitting tend to have 'spreading'

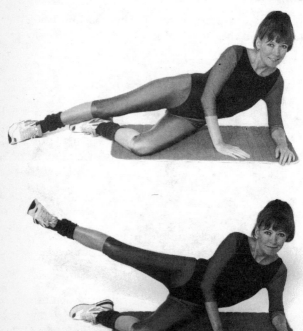

bottoms, hips and thighs. We aim to tighten everything in with some deep-muscle work. You can literally take inches off with the right contouring exercises.

Side leg raises are a common exercise, but often carried out wrongly so that the part you think you're exercising is hardly working at all. This time let's do it right. Lie on your left side, supporting your upper body weight on your left forearm and right hand as shown, with your left leg bent and your hips facing directly forwards. Your tummy should be tucked in. Now raise your right leg, without locking the knee, to 45 degrees. Keep the knee facing forwards, foot facing forwards and hips square to the front.

Raise and lower the leg slowly 10 times.

Turn over and repeat on the other side for a complete set. Do a Hip Stretch (see page 135) between sets.

Tips

The most common faults are that you tip your top hip back to make the exercise easier and that the moving knee and foot point upwards, too. For maximum hip, outer thigh and bottom workout the leg must be positioned correctly. If you prefer, you can lie with your upper body on the floor.

Improving

You can raise the leg up further as long as you don't tip back. You can also do the movement slower.

Super

Do the exercise as before, but split each leg raise into two, or even three, distinct moves. Raise up a few inches (cm), stop; raise up a few more inches; stop. When lowering the leg, do the same. If you are doing more sets,

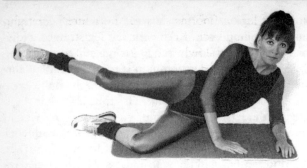

pause in between and stretch out the working hip by bringing the upper knee to rest in front of your body.

Exercise 8: Lower Leg Raises

Standard

This is the best exercise to firm up and contour your inner thighs. Done correctly, it can also work your hips and bottom.

Lie on your left side, head supported on bent or outstretched left arm, right hand on floor in front of you

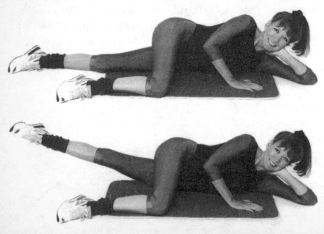

and right leg on floor as shown. Make sure your right hip isn't rolling back. Keep your left leg straight. Now raise your left leg slowly and lower it again to the floor.

Repeat 10 times. Turn over and repeat 10 times on the other leg.

Tips

Don't be surprised if you find it nearly impossible to raise your lower leg even a couple of inches (5 cm) off the floor to begin with! These are seriously neglected muscles in most people, unless you happen to ride horses regularly. Feel the lower hip working in conjunction with the lower leg.

Improving

In time, you'll raise that leg a little higher.

Super

Do the sequence as before, but this time when you raise the lower leg, make the movement into an 'L' by bringing the leg back as far as it will go once it is raised, then bring it back to start. This works the hip and bottom even more. If doing more sets, stretch out your inner thigh by lying on your back with feet almost together, knees bent, and bringing your thighs out to the sides.

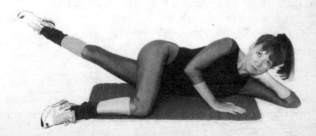

Exercise 9: Bottom Squeezes

Standard

You probably don't need to lose a lot of weight off your bottom, but simply firm and neaten it up. No diet can do that: your bottom needs hard work to return to its natural, firm, rounded shape. The next three exercises will do just that. First, lie on your back with knees bent, feet hip-width apart, hands on chest and pelvis in correct position. Now concentrate on your bottom. Squeeze it together as hard as you can, lifting if off the

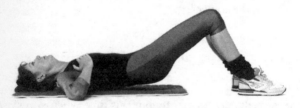

floor slightly.

Hold each squeeze for a couple of seconds and repeat 10 times. Do a Hip Stretch (see page 135) between sets.

Tips

If your bottom muscles are sadly under-used, you may find that little happens when you try to squeeze on the first day or two. Don't let this bother you. Keep concentrating and you'll soon remind the muscles they are there.

Improving

Squeeze harder, squeeze for longer. Practise squeezing throughout the day whenever you remember. (You can squeeze sitting or standing up.)

Super

Start in standard position, raise your right leg straight into the air, then lift and squeeze as before. The raised leg means your bottom has to work harder

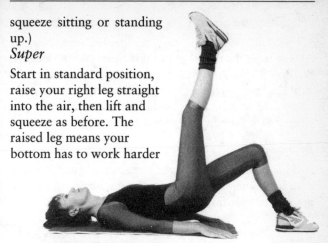

to squeeze itself off the floor.

Exercise 10: Single Leg Raises

Standard

Roll over and lie on your tummy with your head on your hands. Now lift your right leg up and feel the upper hamstring (back of thigh) and bottom working.

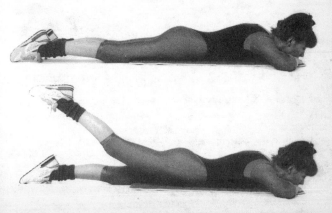

Do 10 raises on the right leg then repeat with the left.

Tips

Aim to relax the rest of your body as you do the leg raises. Stop if your lower back causes you discomfort; you could be raising your leg too high. Lower it a little. Build up to a full set by completing half sets. Finish the sets with a Back Stretch (see page 136).

Improving

Hold each lift a little longer rather than trying to raise your leg higher. Make sure you're not using your hip to pivot your leg off the floor.

Super

Add ankle weights to the standard exercise. If you don't have ankle weights, make small circles with each leg each time you raise it, clockwise then anti-clockwise. Be sure to keep the raised leg straight.

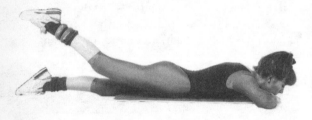

Before further sets do the Back Stretch (see page 136).

Exercise 11: Kneeling Squeezes

Standard

Kneel with your upper body resting on your lower arms as shown. Keep your back flat and tummy pulled in. Now raise your right leg slowly until it is just past parallel to the floor and feel your buttock working. Hold it

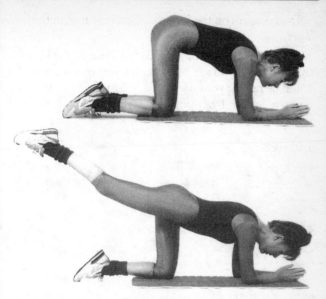

for a second then slowly lower it to the floor.

Repeat 10 times, and then repeat with your left leg.

Do a Back Stretch (see page 136) between sets.

Tips

Don't fling your leg upwards or try to force it past the optimum position. Be careful not to let your lower back sag.

Improving

Concentrate on feeling a really strong, controlled pull along your upper hamstring and in the bottom. The slower you can do these, the better.

Super

Start on all fours as in standard. Lift your right leg to

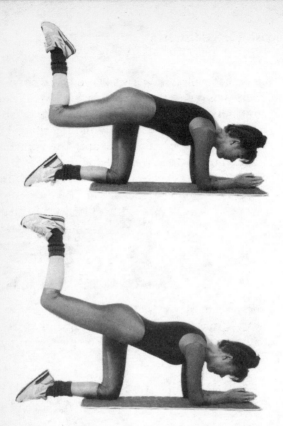

your back, bending the knee, until it is in the position shown. Now slowly lift the bent leg a few inches further, until you feel a deep squeeze in the buttock. Hold for a second, relax and repeat 10 times. Repeat with your other leg.

Arch back up like a cat to finish, and release your lower back.

Exercise 12: Side Stretch

Standard

To achieve the smallest waist possible you need not only to tone the muscles of that area, which we've already done now, but also to elongate them – literally stretching out the area between the pelvis and the ribcage to contour you into a nice hourglass shape. This combination of a side stretch and bend will do that.

Stand with your legs approximately 2 ft (60 cm) apart with your pelvis in correct alignment. Taking care to keep your spine from twisting, bring your left arm up as shown, drop your right arm down your right leg and

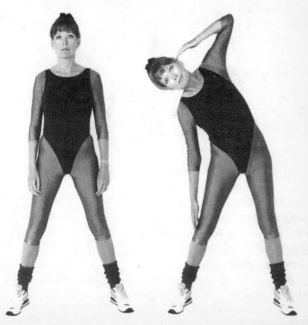

bend to the right, feeling the stretch along the left side.

Return to start and bend to the left side.

Do 10 movements to left and right.

Tips

Do the movement slowly and keep your head facing forward and your neck in alignment with your spine.

Improvement

Hold each stretch a little longer and gradually feel your bend getting deeper.

Super

A similar exercise to standard, but this time when bending to the right, bring your left arm up and over your head to 'lead' your body further into the stretch. Your legs will need to be a little wider apart for this one.

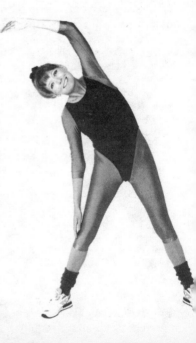

NOTE: If you are doing spot reducing exercises after your body contouring, do them now, before your cool-down.

——BODY CONTOURING——
THE COOL-DOWN

The Hip Stretch

Lie on your back and cross your left leg over your right knee as shown. Clasp your right thigh with your hands and gently and slowly pull it in towards your chest until you feel the optimum stretch in
your left buttock and hip.

Hold for 10 seconds.
Release and repeat to

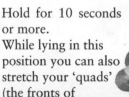

other side.

The Stomach Stretch

Lie on your stomach, as shown, with
arms out in front of you. Now lift up
your head and chest until you feel
the stretch from chest to hips.

Hold for 10 seconds
or more.
While lying in this
position you can also
stretch your 'quads'
(the fronts of

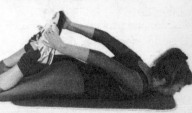

135

your thighs).
Bring your
hands back
to clasp your feet in towards your bottom. Feel the
stretch down the front of each thigh.

The Back Stretch

Kneel on all fours and curl up your spine, then release it
down. Now slowly slide back until you're sitting on
your heels, with your chest touching your knees, your
back and shoulders stretched and your arms out in front

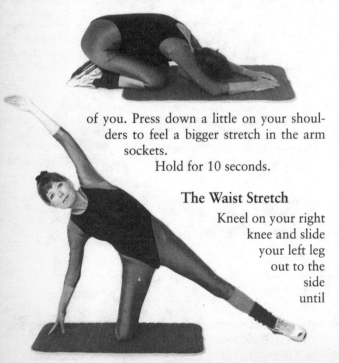

of you. Press down a little on your shoulders to feel a bigger stretch in the arm
sockets.

Hold for 10 seconds.

The Waist Stretch

Kneel on your right
knee and slide
your left leg
out to the
side
until

it is straight. Balance your upper-body weight on your right, your hand placed out to your right side, lifting your left arm

up and over your head towards the right. Hold when you feel a good stretch all along your left side. Your right knee should remain at right angles to the floor. Your spine should remain straight, not twisted to the back or front.

Hold for 10 seconds. Repeat to the other side.

The Triceps Stretch

Stand with a straight back, maintaining the Pelvic Tilt. Raise your right arm up above your head and bend your elbow so that your right hand falls, palm inwards, on to your upper back.With your left hand, clasp the right arm just behind the elbow and gently pull it so that the right hand slides further down the back over towards the left shoulder blade.

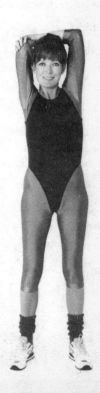

Hold the optimum stretch for 10 seconds, then repeat on the other side.

The Groin Stretch

Sit down with your back straight and the soles of your feet together, about 1 ft (30 cm) in front of you, knees

137

apart. Making sure your
lower back isn't curved, and
your tummy isn't protruding,
lean forwards slightly to
grasp the inside of each ankle
with each hand. Using the
weight of your elbows, gently
press your legs downwards
until you feel a good stretch
in the groin.

Hold for 10 seconds.

The Hamstring Stretch

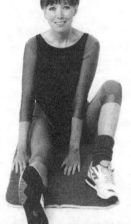

Now release your legs.
Bend your left leg, put
your left foot flat on the
floor and stretch your
right leg out straight
in front of you, again
making sure your
lower back doesn't slump.
(If it does, you may find
doing the exercise with your
back against a wall helps. It
is more important to get a
strong lower back in this
stretch than it is to keep your
leg straight.)

Once your right leg is
straight, lean as far forward
over the leg as you can,
keeping the lower back
strong. You can place your hands lightly on the floor
at either side of your right leg.

Chapter 3
SPOT REDUCING

Is there a particular part of your body that you've always disliked? Your saggy bottom? Your spreading hips? Those jodhpur thighs? A non-existent waist or a flat chest? Every one of us has our own pet hate about our bodies, and while the body-contouring programme concentrates on our whole, now we spend a little 'extra time' on our own particular problem areas.

In this chapter you'll find four different sets of spot reducing exercises to work on the four areas that are the most frequent 'trouble spots'. These exercises re-shape and reduce either by tightening or by elongating the muscles underlying the problem area, while your diet removes the surplus fat as well.

All you need to do is pick which one (if you like, you can pick more than one) you need most and add the routine to your activity programme at least four times a week, as instructed in the 21-day schedule in Chapter 1.

Each routine takes approximately five minutes, and, as you will be adding it on to the end of your body contouring programme or your fat burning programme before the cool-down, there's no need to spend extra time warming up or cooling down.

Variations

You can, if you like, do the programme more than four days a week, but don't attempt the exercises all seven days a week. Five – or, at the most, six – is maximum. All muscles need a day off when you're working them hard, after being under-used for perhaps years!

If you have two particular problem spots, but don't want to add a whole ten minutes on to your exercise routine, you could split them and do one spot reducing programme on two days of the week, and the other on the other two.

However, it is important never to do them in isolation, as your body won't be warm. Always tag them on to the end of contouring or fat burning.

Before you begin

Remember that all the notes that apply to the body contouring chapter also apply here. Read the instructions carefully; carry out the exercises using the proper technique. And keep thinking effort, control, concentration. That's just what's needed ... then the exercises will really work for you.

——SPOT REDUCING ROUTINE 1—— BUST, CHEST AND UPPER BACK

A small or droopy bust can be vastly improved with exercises to straighten an upper back made weak, perhaps, by years of study or desk work, and to stretch and strengthen the chest and pectoral muscles. The actual breast tissue has no muscle in it, but the look and line of the bust can nevertheless be vastly improved (see also the body-awareness section in Chapter 5).

1 The Chest Stretch

Stand with your legs hip-width apart and knees slightly bent. Hold yourself in the correct pelvic tilt. Lift up from your bottom to elongate your spine; keep shoulders down and relaxed, and neck neither poked forward nor pulled back.

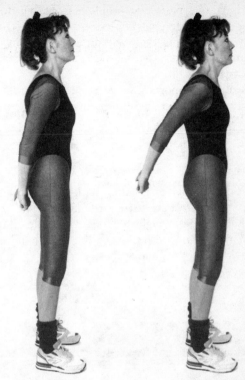

Now clasp your hands behind your back, keeping your arms virtually straight. As you straighten your arms, you will feel your chest 'expand' and your shoulders stretch.

Now, keeping palms facing downwards, pull your arms out as far to the back as they will go, as shown. The pull and stretch across your chest and shoulders will get stronger.

Hold the furthest point for a count of 5 then return to start and repeat up to 10 times.

141

Tips

It is important not to let your neck and shoulders hunch up into your head in this one. Breathe normally throughout.

Improving

As you practise, your arms will go out further and further behind you. If you have a mirror, stand sideways on and check your progress.

2 Arm Lifts

Now lie on your back on the floor with your knees bent, maintaining a correct pelvic tilt throughout the exercise. Take a 3 lb (1.5 kg) weight (or filled vegetable-oil bottle) in each hand and, with elbows bent, bring hands and then elbows in to meet above chest.

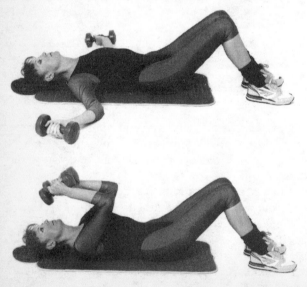

Hold there for a count of 5, return slowly to the floor and repeat 10 times.

Tips

You can start off with lighter weights, or no weights at all, for the first few days. Keep your lower back firmly in place on the floor throughout.

Improving

You can use heavier weights when the 3 lb (1.5 kg) weights start to feel easy, but never go over 5lb (2.5 kg) weights.

3 Standing Shoulder Presses

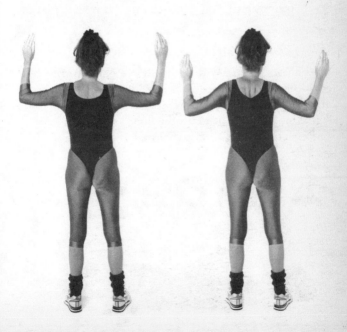

143

Stand as shown, with your legs hip-width apart, knees 'soft' and spine straight, lifting arms up and to sides. Now in one strong movement, pull both elbows down and to the back so that your shoulder blades press together at the end of the movement.

Hold that press for a count of 5, then return and repeat 10 times.

Tips

This helps rid you of the 'salt-cellar' look across your collarbone. Avoid tucking your head and neck forward as you do the movement.

Improving

Keep trying until you can get those shoulder blades together.

4 Lying Arm Raises

Lie on your tummy with your legs straight and arms out in front of you, as shown. Now lift your right arm as high as it will go, and slowly lower. Repeat with your left arm. Lift your head off the floor as you go.

Repeat 10 times with each arm.

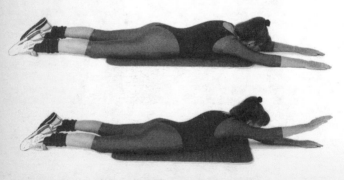

Tips

A slightly easier version is to bend your elbows and raise the arms with your hands just under your chin. Don't be tempted to try arm raises with your head kept on the floor; this doesn't work the right area.

Improving

Try and get the lift higher as you progress. Wear wrist weights for added resistance.

5 Double Press-Ups

Kneel on all fours in the press-up position, keeping your back flat and tummy tucked in. Now do press-ups as you did in the contouring routine, but this time stop

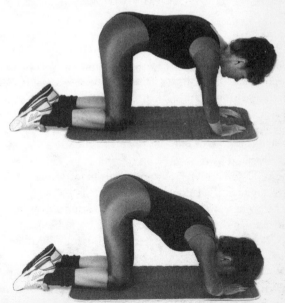

halfway down, pause for a count of 1, then continue to the floor. Stop again halfway up, count 1, and continue back to start. Repeat 10 times.

Tips

Don't forget to keep your tummy in as you go.

Improving

Move your knees further back to make the work more strenuous.

——SPOT REDUCING ROUTINE 2——
STOMACH AND WAIST

If you have a flabby tummy and/or a thick waist, your lifestyle probably has even more to answer for than it does regarding the rest of your body shape. We spend so much of our lives sitting at desks, in cars and in comfy chairs, squashing and shortening and weakening our middles. The middle body, between the lower ribs and the pelvic floor, depends totally upon muscles to keep it in place, and these muscles get very little use in our normal lives. So as time goes on our waistlines literally disappear. Women have the added problem of pregnancy, too, which can weaken the 'abdominals'.

The waist area needs stretching out to counteract thickening; the sides of the waist need tightening, and the abdomen itself needs strengthening for a middle you can easily fit into a size 12 or less.

But there is one bit of good news: the middle body area is the quickest of all to show good results. So get working now!

1 Double Curl-Ups

Lie in the starting curl-up position, knees bent, pelvis tilted correctly, hands lightly on back of head, elbows out. Now curl up, breathing out, but this time do it in two stages, stopping halfway to pause for a count of 1. Return, again stopping halfway for a count of 1.

Repeat 10 times.

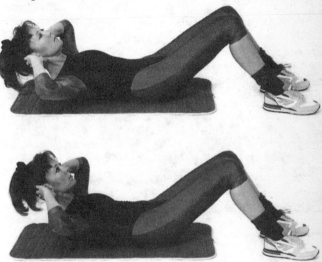

Tips

Remember to keep a good distance between your chin and chest, and to look towards the ceiling, not at your knees.

Improving

For harder work, pull your legs in to your chest as you curl up.

2 Rotated Curl-Ups II

Lie on your back to start, as in the previous exercise. Now raise both legs into a low 'cycling start' position. Raise your left shoulder off the floor and rotate towards your right knee, as you do so bringing your right leg in and breathing out. As you return to the floor, your left leg moves back to start.

Repeat on your left side, doing 10 of these rotations/cycles on each side.

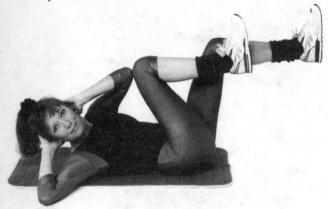

Tips

Your feet shouldn't touch the floor at all throughout this exercise.

Improving

Once your stomach muscles get strong you can speed up this exercise so that your head hardly touches the floor between left and right side moves. Don't let the knee that isn't working on alternate moves fall back out towards the floor, which could strain your lower back. Keep it more or less directly above your hips.

3 Curl-Backs

Sit on the floor with your knees bent, back straight and pelvis correctly tilted. Lift your arms straight out in front of you; breathe in. Breathing out, slowly curl backwards to 45 degrees. Hold for a count of 5 and slowly curl back up.

Repeat 5 times.

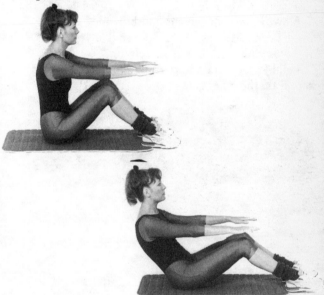

Tips

You may not be able to curl back far at first without your stomach trembling or bulging. If it does either of those, stop and curl back slightly less the next time. There's no point in curling back further than 45 degrees as virtually all the abdominal work is done in the first 45 degrees.

149

Improving

Building up to 10 repeats and/or hold for a count of 10.

4 The Crossed Curl

Lie on your right side with your hips square to the front, and your left foot resting just in front of your right ankle, both arms resting lightly in front of your stomach.

Now, in one movement and breathing out, lift your head, neck and arms off the floor so that your arms slide towards your back over your left hip.

Hold for 5, relax and repeat 10 times. Turn over and repeat on the other side

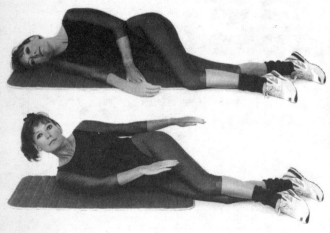

Tips

Look in the direction you're moving. Don't let your left hip slide backwards as you come up.

Improving

Get your shoulders off the floor, too.

5 Alternate Leg Lifts

Lie on your back on the floor, your knees bent and pelvis correctly tilted. Rest hands lightly on either side of your lower stomach. Now, keeping your knee bent, raise your right leg off the floor and bring it in towards your chest as shown.

Then bring your left leg in. Return your left foot to the floor, then slowly return your right foot. On the next repeat, bring your left leg in first, then right leg, then right leg down first, and so on. This exercise works the lower abdomen.

Tips

Use your fingers to feel your lower abdominals working while your legs move.

Improving

Wear ankle weights to make the exercise harder.

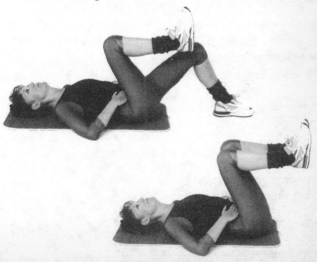

——SPOT REDUCING ROUTINE 3—— BOTTOMS

Yet again a sedentary lifestyle is the major culprit when it comes to bottoms that sag, flag, flatten and generally let you down when it comes to looking nice in a clingy dress.

But a nice, firm, rounded bottom isn't just a vanity; the muscles that give a good 'bun' (as the Americans call it) its shape also help you to stand correctly, supporting the lower back and encouraging the stomach to tuck in. So your bottom can affect your shape in more ways than you probably realized.

Most bottom exercises also work, to some degree, the hips.

1 Sitting Bottom Lifts

Sit on the floor with your legs crossed in front of you, supporting your body weight on your arms behind you as shown, and keeping your back straight. Leaving your ankles on the floor, raise your bottom and squeeze for a count of 5.

Return to start position and repeat 10 times.

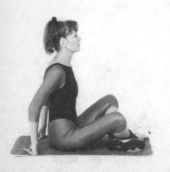 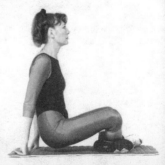

Tips

Concentrate on raising yourself by using your bottom rather than putting too much force on your wrists. If you lean back, the exercise becomes easier, so concentrate on keeping your back at right angles to the floor, or even leaning slightly forwards.

Improving
Hold each lift for longer; lift higher.

2 Lying Bottom Lifts

Lie on your back on the floor, your knees bent, arms by your sides, your feet hip-width apart. Lift your bottom off the floor until your thighs and abdomen are in line. Now open and close your thighs as far as they will go, 20 times.

Relax for 5 seconds then repeat.

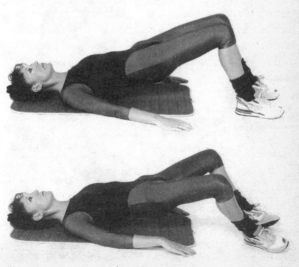

Tips

Put some real effort into this; it's not as easy as it sounds.

Improving

Aim to open the thighs wider, and close them slower.

3 Kneeling Bottom Lifts

Kneel, as shown, with your hands clasped behind your bottom. Now bend forward from the hips until your head touches the floor. Then, using your bottom muscles, pull yourself back up to start. Repeat 20 times.

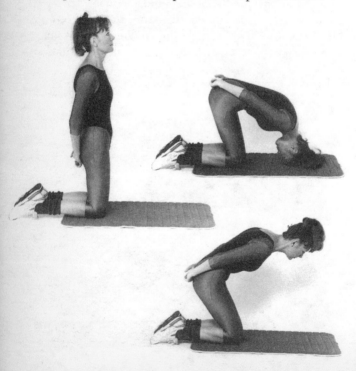

Tips

You should feel your left and right buttocks pulling in as you come up on this. Concentrate on pivoting your upper body and keeping your legs still. Make sure to keep your tummy tucked in throughout.

Improving

Come up in double or treble movements, stopping then starting again.

4 Kneeling Leg Lifts

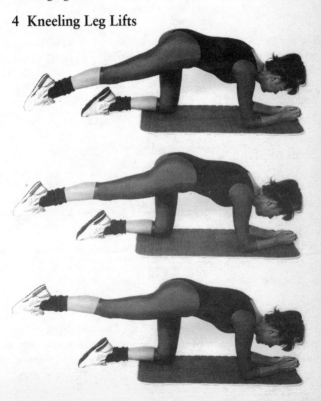

Kneel on all fours, resting your upper body on your fore-arms. Keep your tummy tucked in and your back flat in the correct pelvic position. Now lift your right leg out to the back in a triple movement. Stop a few inches off the floor, count 1, continue a few more inches and count 1, then move to leg parallel with floor position.

Count 1 and repeat as you lower the leg back down to the floor and in to kneeling. Do 5 repeats on your right leg, then repeat the exercise with your left leg.

Tips

Do the movement in a very controlled way, making sure to keep both hips level with the floor. Try to ensure that your lower back doesn't sag.

Improving

You could wear ankle weights to do this exercise.

5 Sit to Stand

Sit near the edge of a sturdy dining-type chair without arms. Have lower legs at right angles to thighs and feet firmly on the floor, a little under hip-width apart. Have your arms loosely at your sides.

Without using your arms, simply come up out of the chair to a standing position.

Sit back down and repeat 20 times.

Tips

The only way you will get out of the chair is to use your bottom and stomach muscles together. At first you may find this exercise totally baffling. Persist; it simply means your bottom and stomach muscles are in even worse condition than you realized!

Improving

Don't move your feet at all. Concentrate on a solid, balanced movement. The further away from the chair you move your feet while in the start position, the harder the exercise will be. (Conversely, the nearer in to the chair your feet are, the easier the exercise is; so don't cheat and get up that way!)

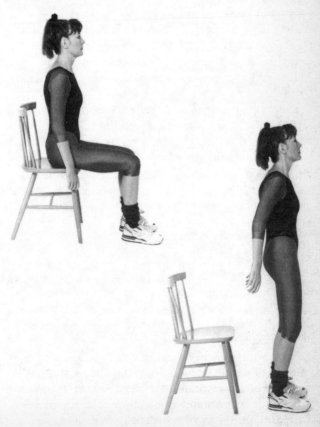

——SPOT REDUCING ROUTINE 4——
HIPS AND THIGHS

British women have a natural tendency to a pear shape; but, again, too many hours sitting rather than standing or walking can have a dire effect, so you mustn't totally blame your genes!

Hips and thighs that sit a lot, spread a lot. They need pulling back into a tight shape with the right exercises. It is sometimes hard to separate hip exercises from ones that also do the bottom good, so these five exercises that follow will also work on the bottom to a lesser degree too.

Exercising the thighs also helps to rid you of dimpled fat in that area, sometimes called cellulite. In fact, in my experience, it is only targeted exercise in this area that will completely rid you of this particularly unattractive fat layer – combined, of course, with a fat burning diet, such as the 21-day regime. If you don't believe me, find me a full-time exercise instructor who has cellulite on her thighs!

1 Standing Hip Lift

Get a chair and stand with your left side towards its back, lightly holding the chair for support. Do a Pelvic Tilt and move your right leg an inch or two (2¹/2–5 cm) off the floor so that your right knee is touching the inside of your left knee as shown.

Now bring your right leg up and back, keeping your knee slightly bent, as far as you can, until you feel your hip and bottom working.

Slowly lower to starting position and repeat 10 times. Turn around and work your left leg in the same way.

Tips

Keep your hand on the hip of the working leg to stabilize the hip, and to get more work into the movement.

Improving

Do two sets and/or add ankle weights.

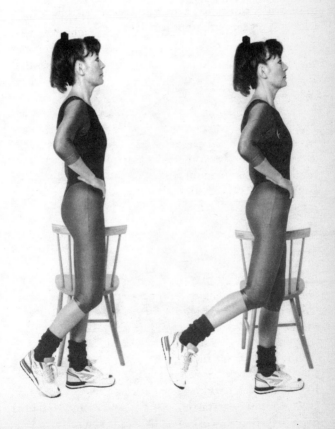

2 Resisted Leg Raises

Lie on your left side with your upper body supported on the left forearm and your right hand placed in front of you. Making sure your hips are square to the front, bend your right leg and place your right foot on top of your left knee, as shown.

Now raise your left leg off the floor, using your right foot to offer resistance. Lower and repeat 10 times. Turn over and repeat with right leg.

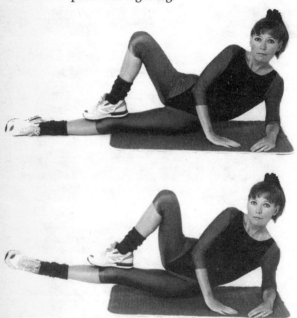

Tips

You may find this exercise easier if you lie stretched full out rather than supporting yourself on your arm.

Improving

Offer more resistance to the movement by exerting more
pressure from your upper foot.

3 Thigh Squeezes

Lie on your back with your knees bent and in correct
pelvic position, and your feet just an inch or two (2¹/₂–5
cm) apart. Now slide your thighs open as far as they will
go, so that the soles of your feet are almost touching.
Keeping your arms relaxed on the floor, bring your
thighs up in a strong movement and squeeze them
together.

At the same time, lift your head off the floor in a mini
curl-up. Really feel your thighs and bottom working.
Repeat the squeeze 20 times.

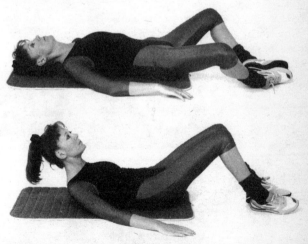

Tips

It is important to keep your back flat and firmly on the
floor throughout this movement.

Improving

The exercise is also good for groin mobility, so don't forget to start with your thighs as wide as you can.

4 Foot Rotations

This is a superb exercise for bringing jodhpur thighs back into line and for tightening wide hips. Lie on your left side with your upper body supported on your left forearm and your right hand in front of you, and with your lower leg bent. Keeping your hips square to the front, raise your right leg as far as it will go, then rotate the ankle and foot clockwise (i.e., up).

Slowly lower and repeat the leg raise and rotation 10 times. Turn over and repeat on the other side.

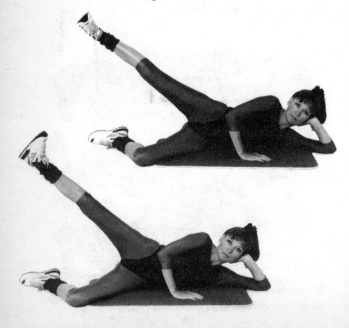

Tips

It is important to keep the foot flexed, the leg straight
and the knee facing forwards. Don't let the upper hip
roll back. When you rotate the ankle you should feel it
in the working hip.

Improving

As you progress, you will rotate the ankle further.

5 Knee and Toe Taps

Lie on your left side with your upper body placed as for
the foot rotations or supported on forearm as shown,
with your left leg slightly bent and your right leg placed
behind the left leg as shown. Now bring your right knee

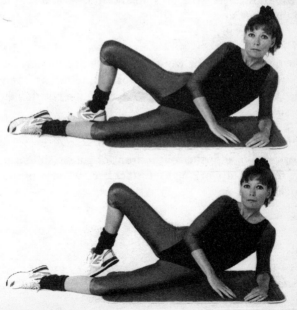

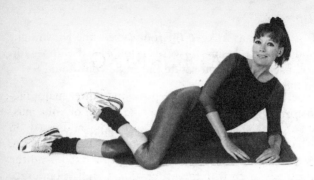

over your left leg to touch the floor in front, then take it back again so your right toe touches the floor behind your leg.

Do 10 of these knee taps, then turn over and repeat on the other side.

Tips

When you bring your working leg back, it is important to keep the hips from swinging back, and the working knee should be brought back to as upright a position as possible.

Improving

Work the knee further out in front of your resting leg; aim to get your working leg further back when your toe touches.

Chapter 4
FAT BURNING

Your shape and your size depend upon three major factors. The first is the size, tone and length of your muscles, problems which we've already addressed in Chapters 2 and 3. The second is your natural skeleton, which, by the time you are an adult, is fixed. And the third has to do with the proportion and distribution of the fat layers in your body. It is this body fat that we are going to tackle here, through special fat burning exercises.

But first, let's look at your body fat in a bit more detail. Most people realize that if they are overweight, much of their surplus weight is fat. A classic size-12 woman of average height with 36-inch (91 cm) hips will probably have around 22 per cent body fat. If she weighs, say, 9 stone (57.1 kg), then she will be carrying about 27 lbs (12.3 kg) of fat. If she's a stone (6.4 kg) heavier – and probably a size 16 – that extra stone (6.4 kg) in weight will be nearly all extra fat. She will carry 41 lbs (19 kg) of fat, which is nearly 30 per cent of her total body weight. And that's nearing the definition for clinical obesity.

This high proportion of body fat can be eliminated in two ways: by diet (like the 21-day diet in Chapter 1), and by exercise. But the right exercise has another special benefit, too. Dieting alone cannot remove fat specifically from where you want it to be lost. For instance, if your thighs are carrying most of the fat, on a normal low-calorie diet they may be the last to show results because, left to its own devices, weight tends to come off from your top downwards. But new research from America backs up what I have found – that if you work the body aerobically, the fat is more likely to go from those stubborn lower body areas where most fat is usually stored on women. One likely explanation for this is that during aerobic exercise the increased metabolic rate of the body manifests itself as greatly increased body heat, which is why you feel so warm when you exercise energetically. Much of this heat is generated by the hard work that the muscles perform. In aerobic exercise, the muscles that do the most work are those of the legs, hips and behind. This increased heat and the prolonged local intense muscle movement in the lower body may actually mobilize the fat stores in those areas and encourage the body to use that fat for energy. Another reason may simply be that the increased oxygen flow to the lower body during exercise increases its capacity to burn fat.

To summarize: the right exercise is important to your re-shaping programme in two ways. It will help you to lose weight by burning up fat, and it will help you to burn up fat more quickly from your problem areas.

What is fat burning exercise?

In order to get your body burning fat for fuel (energy), you must do some continuous exercise over a period of time. If, instead, you exercise in short bursts, say, a run for a bus, a five-minute weight-training session, or a run up a flight of stairs, your body's main source of energy will not be fat, but glycogen. Glycogen is a form of glucose mixed with water and stored in the liver and muscles as a source of immediate energy.

But if you continue to exercise steadily so that your heart rate increases and your intake of oxygen increases – and those increases are sustained – gradually your body begins to use its own fat for fuel. And the use of glycogen then decreases. As the table on page 169 indicates, the amount of fat you burn begins to exceed the amount of glycogen you're burning after 15 minutes of exercise. At around the 40-minute point, your fat burn is at its maximum.

Surprisingly enough, the best fat-burning exercise isn't the exercise that has you puffing and panting hardest and that causes your muscles to ache. The best is what is called 'low-intensity' aerobic exercise. This needs explaining.

Aerobic exercise is exercise that raises your heart rate to between 60 per cent and 85 per cent of its maximum. Low-intensity aerobic exercise stays at around the lower level, 60–70 per cent. This is the level at which you're breathing harder than normal and feel you are working quite hard. But you should still be able to talk and you shouldn't feel uncomfortable. The level of work is one that you can sustain without continually stopping to recover.

As your lungs breathe in more deeply, they are taking in more oxygen, which is absolutely vital to the fat-burning process. Without oxygen your body cannot burn up its own body fat. And the raised heartbeat means the heart is working harder to get that oxygen to your muscles via the bloodstream.

As the days and weeks go by and you continue your fat-burning programme, your lungs and heart become more efficient and can provide even more oxygen for the fat-burning fire. And that means you burn even more fat.

——THE 21-DAY FAT BURNING——
PROGRAMME

What I, and many experts, consider to be the best form of fat burning exercise is walking. Walking is by far the easiest way to maintain a steady low-intensity workout. It is also possible – and immediate – for nearly everyone; is low in cost and should be enjoyable. Therefore, the 21-day Schedule in Chapter 1 includes a five-times-a-week graduated walking programme as your fat burning activity.

By its very nature, walking tends to be a low-intensity workout, but if you are a beginner, it is useful to be able to check whether or not you are in the 60–70 per cent heart rate range while you walk. For this you need to check the following chart, and then take your pulse for 10 seconds from time to time during your walk session.

When you have done this on a few occasions, you will soon be able to link up how you feel with your probable pulse rate. At the 60 per cent level, you should feel that you are working hard but that you can still talk, and that you have no urge to stop and rest. A word of caution, though: if you feel little or no exertion, you are probably below the 60 per cent level and won't be achieving a real fat burning 'walkout' at all.

Taking your pulse

Place the first and second finger of your right hand on the pulse spot of your neck – just below the centre of the right jawline. Using a watch with a second hand, count the beats for 10 seconds. If the rate is slower than the 60–70 per cent rate for your age on the chart, work a little harder; if it is faster, slow down a little.

Don't measure your pulse with your thumb; it has its own pulse which may confuse you. You can also measure your pulse rate in your wrist, but I prefer the neck as the beat is usually much easier to find.

Heart Rate Chart for Optimum Fat Burning

Age	60–70% heart rate per 10 seconds
20 – 25	20 – 23
26 – 30	19 – 22
31 – 35	19 – 22
36 – 40	18 – 21
41 – 45	18 – 21
46 – 50	17 – 20
51 – 55	17 – 20
56 – 60	16 – 19
61 – 66	15 – 18

Glycogen/Fat Burning Ratio Chart

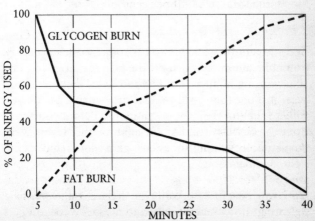

Walking Guidelines

Within the 21-day programme in Chapter 1 you will find (under the 'Your Activities for Today' section each day) specific walking targets in terms of time spent walking and target distance to cover. But here are some general notes to help you get the most from your programme.

Motivation

Fat burning in itself is a big motivation to get walking, but don't forget the other benefits it can bring:

• Fat is burned from the stubborn hip, thigh and bottom areas.
• Muscles are toned in that area, too, plus your stomach is worked.
• Your lung and heart (cardiovascular) fitness is increased. The walking programme will help you to feel fitter and to give you an increased sense of wellbeing.
• Walking is a pleasant way to wind down and ease stress; the ideal relaxation.

Clothing

Wear layers to walk in; you'll soon warm up (a sign you're beginning to burn off the fat). If you go out in a thick woolly jumper you'll be too hot. Likewise, if you wear just one thin T-shirt and shorts when it's cool, you might find – in the cool-down period before you arrive home – you wish you had brought another layer. Wear comfortable walking shoes or jogging shoes and socks.

Accessories

You will benefit, especially on longer walks, from a lightweight rucksack in which to put in layers you peel off, a lightweight waterproof jacket and a drink (from the Unlimiteds list).

Weather

If you wait for perfect walking weather, you won't walk much. So, unless we are talking about thick snow or ice, or thick fog or blizzard conditions, or temperatures over the '80s, get out there and walk!

Time of day

Fit your fat burning plan into your daily routine; but on days when you are also doing the body contouring, try to have a gap of at least a few hours between the two. You won't come to any harm walking either on a fairly empty stomach or after a light meal, but never go thirsty.

Safety

If walking alone, don't forget to bear in mind some points for your own safety:

• Don't walk alone after dark.
• Don't walk in isolated areas.
• Before you go out, tell someone where you are going and roughly how long you're going to be.

Consider walking with a friend for added safety.

Route

It's best either to plan out a route that you know you can walk in the right period of time, or else simply walk out for half your time and walk back the other half. Try to vary your routes for maximum enjoyment. Another idea is to drive to a walk starting point.

Distance

It is more important to walk for the time required in the programme each day, and to maintain your 60–70 per cent heart rate than it is to achieve an exact distance during your walk. However, distance targets are given in the programme and, should you wish, you can measure how far you walk. For this you will probably need a pedometer (available from sports shops). The advantage of measuring distance is that it is a good way of recording your progress. As you get fitter, you will be able to walk faster without raising your heart rate above the 70 per cent level. If you can walk further than the target distances given in the allotted time, then you know you're getting fit!

Walking Style

The right way to conduct your walk is to begin fairly gently and gradually speed up, both by lengthening your stride and by moving your legs faster, until you are at the 60 per cent minimum heart rate. You keep to this pace for the time given in your programme each day, then you gradually slow down the pace until by the time you have finished your walk your heart rate is down to normal, and you have cooled down as you would at the end of a workout. (Check your normal heart rate by taking your pulse – see page 168 – for 10 seconds while you are sitting quietly. An average heart rate for a woman is around 70–80 beats per minute.)

As you get fitter, you can give yourself more work by moving from a brisk stride to an extended stride, and by pumping your arms vigorously. Whatever pace you are walking at, concentrate on good walking posture and a good stride length (see photos, page 175). The pelvic tilt should be maintained as you walk.

Breathing

Breathe evenly and deeply, without making yourself dizzy. Remember, to burn fat, your body needs oxygen!

Exertion

Remember, this is a low-intensity exercise; the idea is to work yourself moderately hard, not to exhaust yourself. If you become breathless, feel unable to talk, feel dizzy, feel any discomfort in your chest or burning or weakness in your thighs or calves, slow down. You are working too hard; the exercise is not aerobic and not doing you any good. If you have a watch with a second hand on you, check your pulse every few minutes if you are at all unsure about whether or not you are working at the right level.

Cool-Down Stretches

When you have finished your walk it is a good idea to do a few leg stretches to help prevent any muscular stiffness the next day. It only takes a minute.

1 *Quad (Front Thigh) Stretch*

Stand (left hand supporting you on the back of a chair, if you like) with your legs together. Bring your right foot up and back, and hold it with your right hand, as shown. Feel the stretch down your thigh.

Hold for a count of 10. Repeat on the other side.

2 *Calf Stretch*

Stand with your right leg approximately 1 ft (30 cm) behind your left leg, both knees bent and with your body weight in between both legs. Press your right heel into the floor, to feel the stretch along the back of your right calf.

Hold for a count of 10. Repeat on the other side.

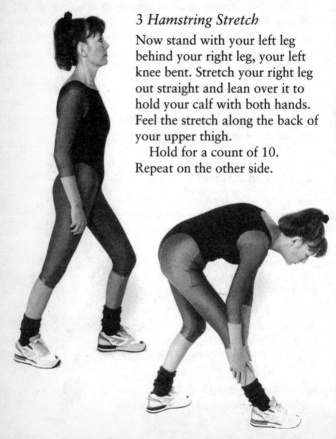

3 *Hamstring Stretch*

Now stand with your left leg behind your right leg, your left knee bent. Stretch your right leg out straight and lean over it to hold your calf with both hands. Feel the stretch along the back of your upper thigh.

Hold for a count of 10. Repeat on the other side.

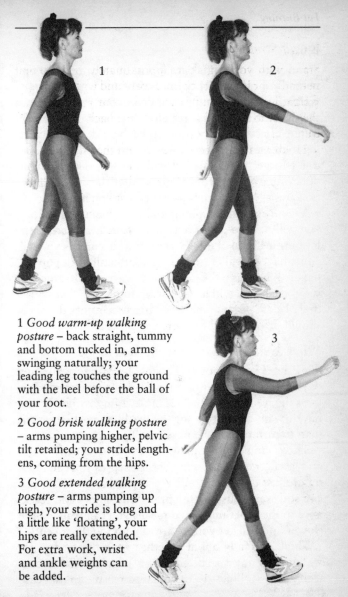

1 *Good warm-up walking posture* – back straight, tummy and bottom tucked in, arms swinging naturally; your leading leg touches the ground with the heel before the ball of your foot.

2 *Good brisk walking posture* – arms pumping higher, pelvic tilt retained; your stride lengthens, coming from the hips.

3 *Good extended walking posture* – arms pumping up high, your stride is long and a little like 'floating', your hips are really extended. For extra work, wrist and ankle weights can be added.

Notes

• Never go into a brisk walk without warming up first with a few minutes of normal walking.

• Uphill walking can be included in the programme as you get fitter. Walking uphill increases the muscle-toning effect on the bottom and calves; downhill walking increases the effect on the thighs and stomach. But don't forget that downhill walking will decrease your pulse rate, so plan your route so that the downhill section comes last and acts as your cool-down.

• As you continue walking and get progressively fitter, you will need to do more to keep your heart rate at the fat burning level of 60–70 per cent. This means you will either have to walk faster in the allotted time, or you will have to increase the workload with uphill work or weights, or you will have to walk for longer. But within the 21-day programme, the suggested times/distances should provide all the progress you need.

What to do if you can't walk today

Sometimes it may not be possible for you to walk on a day that I have listed in your 21-day programme. Perhaps the weather really does make it impossible, or you have to stay in waiting for the washing-machine repair man to turn up, and he never does . . .

There shouldn't be many days when you can't walk; and, as a general rule, most of the excuses you can think up are just that: excuses. Even if you have a baby, you can still walk. Pushing the pram will simply add resistance to the programme and means you can walk a little slower and still get your heart rate up to 60 per cent!

Think carefully about whether your reason for not walking on any specific day is a genuine reason or a feeble excuse. Illness is, of course, a reason. In that case you should suspend the activity programme altogether until you are better.

If you have decided you don't want – or are unable – to walk, well, don't worry. I have devised three simple programmes that will help burn up the fat when you can't get out to walk.

They are not as effective in burning off fat as the walking programme, for the simple reason that they are not as long. But they will help you to maintain cardiovascular fitness so that when you start walking again your lung capacity will not have dropped off. They will also keep your motivation up; they'll keep your lower body in condition for walking and they will, of course, burn up some calories and help to keep your metabolism alive and kicking.

And, if you combine them in one or more of the ways I suggest below, you will burn up plenty of fat, too.

——THE STEPPING PROGRAMME——

Even if you haven't tried stepping, I'm sure you will have heard of it. You step up and off a platform between 6 and 10 inches (15–25 cm) high. Sounds boring, but it needn't be, especially if you step to music. It's worth investing in a step for your home if you are likely to be 'confined to barracks' very often. Less floor space is needed to do a worthwhile step routine than an aerobics dance routine and if bottom, hips and thighs are your trouble spots, stepping is as good as walking for beating that problem.

When you begin stepping, you will find that you – and your legs – get tired quite quickly, so do the routine that follows only as many times as you can manage. The single routine takes about 6 minutes, so if you do it, say, four times, you'll be burning off plenty of fat towards the end.

Stepping tips

• Buy the sturdiest step you can afford; preferably one with adjustable height so you can start off at 6 inches (15 cm) and build up to 10 inches (25 cm).
• Step to music – it makes it much more fun.
• Wear suitable exercise wear plus flexible shoes with a grip sole; aerobic shoes are ideal.
• The routine that follows is a basic step routine. If you get the step bug you could invest in a step video for a more complete aerobic workout.
• Keep leaning into the step when you do the routine.

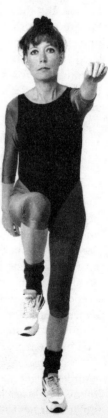

Step Warm-Up

March on the spot for a minute, swinging your arms higher and higher.

Step 1: Basic Step

Stand in front of the step and place your right foot completely on it. Place your left foot on the step. Step down with your right foot, then step down with your left. Continue stepping for 1 minute. Change your lead foot by tapping a beat with your left foot at the end of a sequence and placing it on

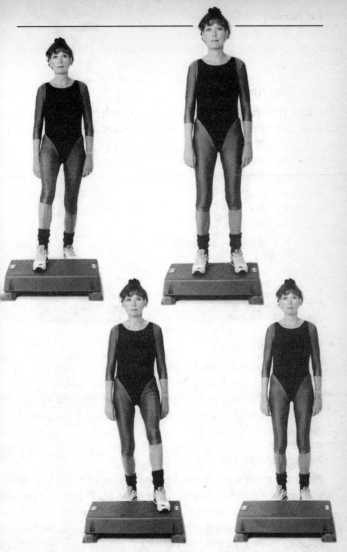

the step first. Follow with your right foot, then step down with your left foot. Then your right.

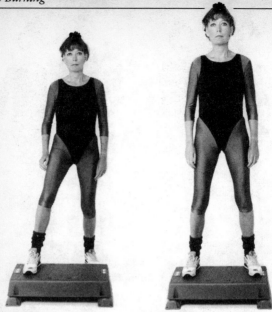

Step 2: Wide Steps

Proceed as you did for the basic step but this time stand with your legs a little more than hip-width apart, and carry out the moves keeping your legs this far apart. Continue for 1 minute; change your lead foot and repeat.

Step 3: Diagonals

The start position is in front of the left corner of the step, with your left hip facing towards the step. Place your left foot on the step towards the left side, then bring your right leg up, rotating your body and your leg so that your right foot places itself on the right edge of the step with the toes pointing inwards towards the middle of the step. As you do so, your left foot moves to the floor at

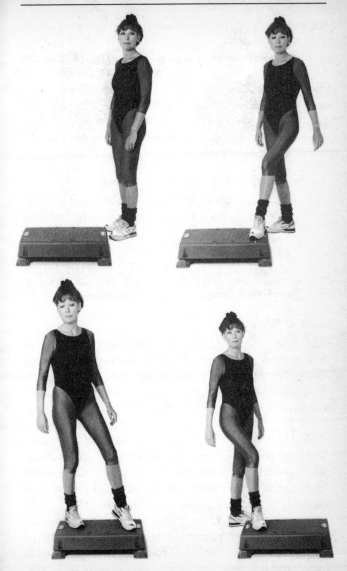

the right base of the step. Your right foot comes off the step to the floor.

The second diagonal repeats the move the opposite way. The right foot is placed on the right side of the step, then your left foot and body are rotated so that your left foot comes down on the left side of the step, with the toes pointing inwards, and your right foot comes off the step, back to its original position at the start of the move. Repeat for 1 minute.

Step 4: Diagonals with Backward Step

Follow the instructions for diagonals, but at the end of each move (i.e., as soon as your left foot has hit the floor on the first diagonal and your right foot has hit the floor on the second diagonal) step backwards with the foot that is left on the step, as shown, for 1 beat. Replace it on the step and continue as before.

Repeat for 1 minute.

Repeat this step sequence as many times as you feel able, then do the cool-down.

Step Cool-Down

March on the spot, as for the warm-up, then do Quad, Calf and Hamstring Stretches as in the walking cool-down. (See Cool-Down Stretches, pages 173–4.)

——THE INDOOR JOGGING—— PROGRAMME

You needn't go outdoors to jog. Jogging on the spot is ideal if you are short of space. I prefer walking to jogging outdoors; but, take my word for it, if you are confined to a small area, it is much more easy and much more rhythmic to jog in a static position than it is to walk on the spot.

As for the stepping programme, you need to wear exercise clothes and some aerobic-type flexible, cushioned shoes.

Jogging Warm-Up

First, start gently walking on the spot, lifting your heels and flexing the balls of your feet, gently swinging your arms. Then march for 1 minute, lifting your knees higher and higher, and swinging your arms higher and higher.

The Jog

Now start jogging. Do as many minutes as you can, up to a maximum of 5 minutes the first day; add on a maximum of 3 minutes each day. End up jogging for as long a period as you like, as long as you feel comfortable.

Remember, the idea is to find a pace that keeps your heart rate raised to low intensity level but no higher, so if you're jogging correctly, you definitely shouldn't feel exhausted after a minute or two.

Slow down the pace by raising your feet less far off the floor, by pumping your arms less and by lifting each leg more slowly. Increase the pace by lifting your feet higher, pumping your arms harder and lifting your legs more quickly.

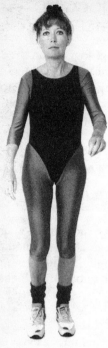 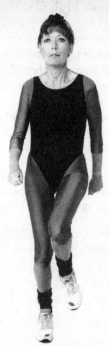

*Slow down the
pace by raising
your feet less*

*Increase the pace
by lifting your
feet higher*

Jogging tips

• If you have a clock or watch with a second hand, measure your pulse occasionally as you would when walking.

• To add interest to the programme – and perhaps to keep you going for longer – you can break up the jog with one or two half-minute step variations. You could choose from one or more of the following:

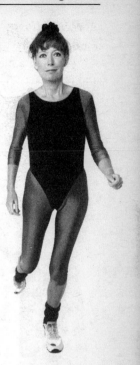

Legs to back. Continue the jogging foot pattern, but as each leg rises, bring it out behind you instead of to the front. Arms should pump to the back as well.

Skips. See Aerobics Move 5, page 189.

Scissors. See Aerobics Move 7, page 90.

Lastly, always jog on the balls of your feet, remember correct pelvic alignment and breathe steadily and as deeply as you can for maximum fat burning.

Jogging Cool-Down

Repeat warm-up sequence in reverse, then do the Quad, Calf and Hamstring Stretches as in the walking cool-down. (See Cool-Down Stretches, pages 173–4.)

——THE AEROBICS PROGRAMME——

Everyone loves to dance, so if you put on some music with a steady beat you can have some real fun with these easy aerobic movements. Put together in a sequence they are designed to warm you up and bring you back down gradually so you feel no strain.

The whole sequence will take about 3 minutes, but once you have mastered it you can repeat Moves 3–7 as many times as you like. Always start your aerobic session with Moves 1 and 2, and finish with Moves 8 and 9, however many times you have repeated Moves 3–7.

185

Aerobics tips

• Wear exercise clothes and aerobic shoes.
• If you find a move makes you breathless, leave it out and just march on the spot or do knee lifts until you are fitter.
• You could mix and match the aerobic, jogging and stepping programmes if you like. Do, say, 5 minutes of each, with one warm-up to start and one cool-down to finish.

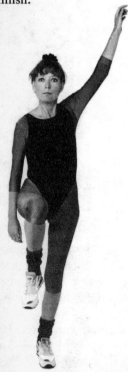

• Check your heart rate if you can during the aerobic session.
• Don't forget to keep your tummy and bottom tucked in.
• Put some real effort into lifting those arms high; raising those knees up.

Aerobics Warm-Up

March on the spot for 1 minute and do large arm circles towards the back.

Aerobics Move 1: Step to the Side and Clap

Take a large step to your right, first with right foot, then left, lift arms and clap as you do so. Then transfer weight and step to the left.

Repeat for 30 seconds.

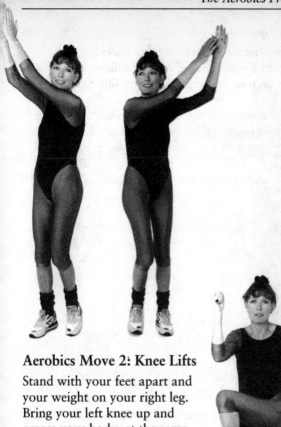

Aerobics Move 2: Knee Lifts

Stand with your feet apart and your weight on your right leg. Bring your left knee up and across your body, at the same time bringing your right elbow down to meet your knee.

Do 10 lifts on the right side; transfer weight to left side and bring right knee up, left elbow down.

Do 10 more lifts. Repeat whole sequence.

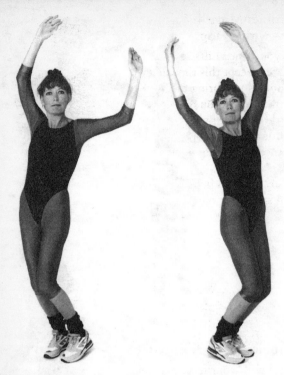

Aerobics Move 3: Twist on the Spot

Keeping your legs together, your knees slightly bent,
raise your arms into the air and twist your whole body
round to the right, then to the left. As you twist to the
right, move your arms to the left – and vice versa – so
that you are working your waist as well as your lower
body.

Repeat, twisting for 30 seconds.

Aerobics Move 4: Knee Lifts with a Hop

Do your Knee Lifts as before, except this time add a hop. As you bring the right knee up, you do a little hop with your left foot. Watch your balance as you go; don't hop too high.
Do 10 lifts and hops on each side, then repeat.

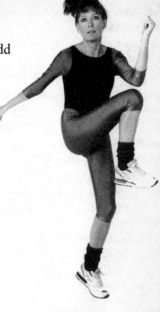

Aerobics Move 5: Skips

Skip on the spot, raising alternate legs to the front and letting arms swing freely as you go. (You know you're skipping correctly when your body feels as light as air and your feet spend a very short time on the floor.) Skip for 1 minute.

Aerobics Move 6: Knee Lifts with a Hop

Repeat Move 4.

Aerobics Move 7: Scissors

Stand with your legs together. Now, as you bring your right leg forward, take your left leg back. In a jumping motion, move so that your left leg is forward and your right leg is back. Your arms should swing as for marching – alternately to your legs.

Jump through 10 scissors movements. March on spot for a count of 10, then jump through 10 more.

Aerobics Move 8: Knee Lifts

Repeat Move 2.

Aerobics Move 9: Step to the Side and Clap

Repeat Move 1.

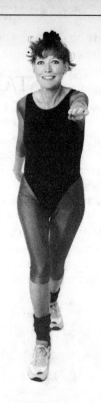

Aerobics Cool-Down

March on the spot for 1 minute, then do the Quad, Calf and Hamstring Stretches, as outlined in the walking cool-down. (See Cool-Down Stretches, pages 173–4.)

Chapter 5
INSTANT SLIMMING
—— THE ART OF BODY AWARENESS ——

How would you like to make yourself look – and measure – slimmer within minutes? Yes, it can be done. It is possible to slim your waist and flatten your stomach; to tighten your bottom and raise your bustline; even to add to your height. And this 'instant slimming' effect is *in addition* to the benefits of your 21-day diet and exercise programme.

Instant slimming is achieved by what I call 'body awareness'; that is, discovering correct body alignment and balance, and then practising this correct alignment throughout the days and weeks ahead so that the 'instant slimming' effect becomes a more permanent reality.

After all, it hardly makes sense to do half an hour or so of exercise a day to improve your shape, only to spend the remaining 23½ hours using your body incorrectly. Doing this actually counteracts the good effect of those exercises.

Yet, that is exactly what many people do. Either through laziness, bad habits or a particular lifestyle, we become a shape we weren't intended to be! By standing incorrectly, sitting incorrectly, walking incorrectly, even lying in bed incorrectly, we weaken certain muscles that should be strong; shorten others that should be long, and tighten muscles that should be flexible. Over the years, these posture problems grow worse, and our shapes grow worse, too.

As a typical example, if you spend years slumped over an office desk, the most visible result is likely to be rounded shoulders and a thickened waist. But the good news is that just as poor body alignment soon gives you a poor body shape, so re-learning correct alignment can soon reverse the problems.

So let's get started – first of all by taking a closer look at just how much effect right – and wrong – body alignment does have on your shape.

Look Slimmer ... Now

For instant slimming you need a full-length mirror, and you need to wear a leotard (or something similar, like a bodysuit, a swimsuit, or briefs and bra). Keep your feet bare, and if you have long hair, fix it up so you can see your shoulders, neck and back.

Now stand sideways to the mirror so you can see your profile in your normal standing posture. (Don't think about this, just stand there as you would when, say, waiting in a queue.) Next, look into the mirror. Do you see anything about your body that resembles the photo here *(Fig. 1)*?

Starting from the top. The *head* pokes forward and so the *chin* lifts high to compensate, squashing the back of the neck in turn. The *shoulders* are slumped forward with shoulder blades sticking out, and as a result the *bustline* has flattened and lowered. The *lower-back* curve is exaggerated, and the *bottom* sticks out to compensate for the imbalance in the upper body. Therefore, the pelvis is tipped forward and the *stomach* protrudes.

All in all, it's a sorry sight!

I'm not saying that you necessarily look like this, but there are very few of us who do have perfect alignment. You may have just one or two of the symptoms, but a

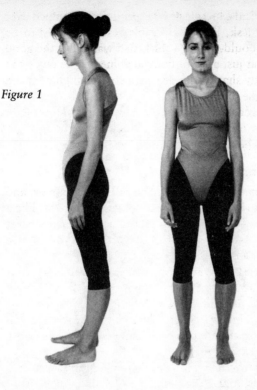

Figure 1

Figure 2

small problem needs working on before it becomes a bigger one.

Now turn around and look at your front view this time *(Fig. 2)*. The profile problems seen from the front show themselves in some or all of the following shape faults. Your *neck* may seem short; your *bustline* may be low; your *waist* may be wide. Travelling down, your *knees* may face slightly inwards (a direct result of weak stomach and bottom muscles, and tight hip flexors and hamstrings). Lastly, you may have flat *foot* arches.

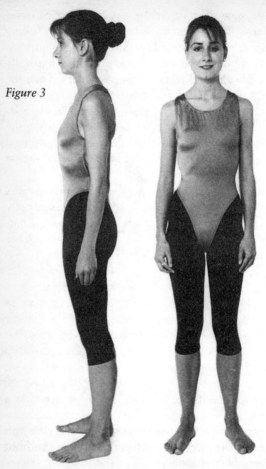

Figure 3

Figure 4

Now, look at the second set of photos here *(Figs 3 and 4)*. It's the same body on the same day. But doesn't that body look better; doesn't it look *slimmer*? How has this happened? All the model is doing is standing correctly balanced and aligned.

194

The side view shows that she has now carried out a correct Pelvic Tilt by slightly softening the knee, pulling in the stomach and hips, and tucking under the bottom. This also lengthens and straightens the spine, naturally lifting the ribcage and relaxing the shoulders. Then the bustline lifts; the neck straightens.

Seen from the front, this all has the effect of elongating the neck, giving the shoulders a better line, widening the gap between waist and bust, slimming the waist itself and correcting the legline. The model will also, almost miraculously, be taller!

In other words, body awareness has instantly created a more shapely figure which will fit much more happily into a smaller dress size, which will look better in whatever is worn, and which will help any dress to hang better.

Try altering your stance now and see the difference for yourself. However, if your poor body alignment is the product of years of bad habits, and you now try to maintain this new alignment for the rest of the day (or even for a quarter of an hour, perhaps!), you may find it hard. This is because, as I explained earlier, misused and disused muscles need working on before you can expect them to perform happily new 'tricks' – albeit the right ones – all day long.

So you actually have to exercise the weakened muscles and stretch the tightened, stiff muscles so that you can maintain the correct alignment easily and without strain throughout the day.

How long this will take depends on how long you've been doing the wrong things, and how bad the problem has become. You've looked at yourself in the mirror, but for a clearer assessment of what, if any, your problems are, try the following movements.

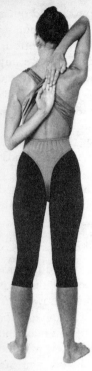

• Stand up straight, raise your right arm and put your left hand behind your body. Can you touch the fingers of both hands together behind your shoulder blades? If they are miles apart, your chest and shoulders need work.

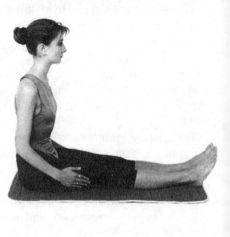

• Sit on the floor with your back straight, your arms at your sides. Can you place both legs in front of you, flat on the floor, without either bending your knees or slumping your back? The more you have to bend your knees, the tighter your hamstrings are, and this means your lower body needs work.

• Can you lie on your back and bring both knees in to touch your chest (using your arms to help, if necessary)? If not, your lower back needs releasing.

• Can you lie on your back on the floor with one leg in to your chest, and keep the other leg straight out on the

196

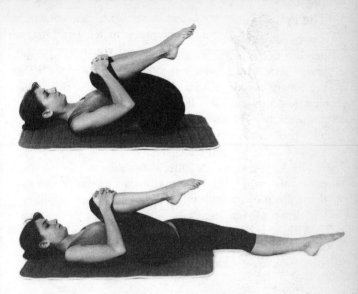

floor? If the straight leg rises off the floor, your hip flex-ors are tight.

If you had trouble with any or all of these test positions, or if you find it hard to maintain a lying pelvic tilt (see page 200), your body alignment is poor and needs some work to maximize all the benefits of the 21-day pro-gramme.

——THE SOLUTION——

First, you have to practise standing, sitting, and lying correctly and you have to work on those muscles that will hold you correctly. Secondly, you have to become 'body aware' throughout your daily life. Let's deal with the first point first.

The Pelvic Tilt

The basis of good body alignment is to learn the correct pelvic tilt. The pelvic bone runs across the whole of your lower body, and supports you, rather like a cup. However, many people stand with their pelvic bone tipped so that the 'cup' is 'spilling forward', rather than upright as it should be. That is why many otherwise slim people have problem tummies. It's normally nothing more than the pelvis not being tilted correctly.

The wrong pelvic posture also leads to lower-back problems and can eventually have repercussions throughout your whole body, right up to your shoulders and down to your feet.

Without the correct pelvic tilt your body can't be well

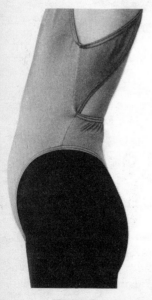
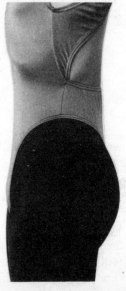

WRONG   RIGHT

balanced and it will change and modify itself to counter-act that incorrect balance. So the very first thing you have to practise doing is a correct pelvic tilt; and that means when standing, sitting, walking . . . all the time.

To practise the tilt, just stand normally. Now tighten your bottom, and pull your stomach 'through to your back' so that your hips lift slightly, your stomach flat-tens out and you feel your torso lengthen. It is not a big movement, just a rocking back into line. If you look at your body's profile in a mirror before you do a correct tilt and while you do a correct tilt, it is easy to see the difference.

Check the sitting pelvic tilt is correct by flattening out your lower back and pulling in your stomach. And the

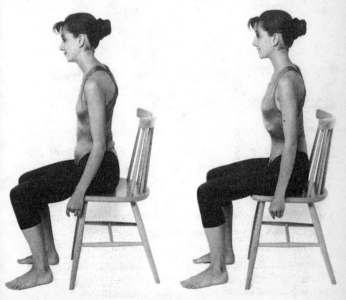

WRONG   RIGHT

lying pelvic tilt can be checked by making sure your lower back is flat on the floor, bed, etc., when your knees are raised. When lying with your legs straight, there will be a slight natural curve in the lower back.

WRONG

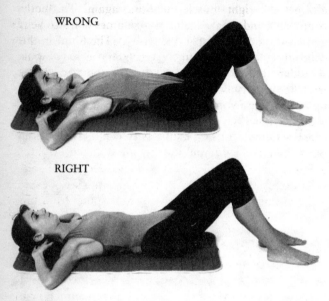

RIGHT

Whenever you stand, you should aim to adopt the correct pelvic tilt, keeping your shoulders relaxed but your spine erect, lifting your ribcage out and up from your waist area. This is the alignment you need to maintain while you walk, swinging from the hips with your knees soft, and your arms swinging softly too.

When you sit, don't cross your legs; keep your back and shoulders aligned as you would for standing. When you go to bed at night, try to sleep with your shoulders relaxed and a 'long' neck, rather than hunching up into a ball.

——THE BODY RE-ALIGNMENT—— PROGRAMME

Practising the right body alignment like this will gradually get the right muscles working again. The body contouring and spot reducing programmes will also help a great deal; for example, Exercise 2 (The Ship) in the contouring section is a fine exercise if you have weak shoulders and a tight chest, and all the cool-down stretches performed regularly will gradually loosen you up and increase your flexibility.

So, if your body alignment is not too bad, then the exercise you are already doing may well be enough to put you on the right track.

But, if your alignment is very poor, you should consider doing some extra work. The following set of exercises works on the most likely 'trouble spots' from top to toe.

I recommend doing this whole routine at least three times a week; it takes about ten minutes. It's better to do the whole routine rather than picking out a couple of exercises for what you consider is your worst area because, as I explained earlier, poor alignment tends to have repercussions throughout the whole body. As an example, a tight, short neck is much more likely to be a symptom of incorrect pelvic tilt and weak back and stomach muscles than it is likely to be a problem on its own. Therefore, if you just work on the neck, the underlying cause remains.

And the other reason is that muscles work in pairs. For example, if your lower back muscles are tight, their opposites – the stomach muscles – will be weak and loose. If your shoulders are weak, your chest muscles are likely to be tight. So you have to work on strengthening

201

one while you loosen up the other.

If you do this programme on its own you will need to warm up and cool down as for any other programme. The body contouring warm-up and cool-down in Chapter 2 are ideal.

For Upper Body

Neck release

Stand with your shoulders as relaxed as you can. Now place the palm of your right hand on the top of your head, just to left of centre, and *gently* bring your neck and head down to the right. Hold for a count of 5. Repeat on the other side.

Now place both palms on the back of your head, towards the top, and gently bring your neck and head forwards and down. Hold for 5 counts.

Shoulder squeeze

Stand, or sit on a stool if you prefer, with the correct pelvic alignment. Clasp your hands behind your back, keeping your elbows bent. Now press your elbows in towards each other, keeping your hands still and your shoulders down. Squeeze as hard as you can, then release and repeat 10 times.

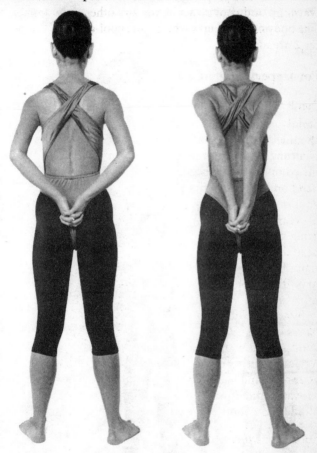

Push-backs

Sitting or standing as before, raise your arms out to the sides to shoulder level. Keeping your pelvis still, push

your arms backwards.
Return to the beginning and
repeat. Start off with 5
repeats and work up to 20.

Elbow push backs

Sit or stand as before and
place the palms of your
hands on your ribcage
below the bust. Now push
your elbows back and in, in
a strong, firm movement.
Then return to the begin-
ning and repeat 20 times.

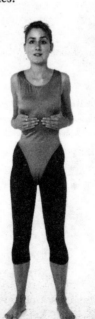

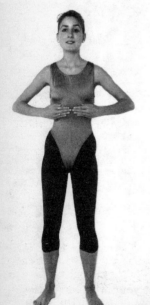

For Pelvic Alignment

Curl-ups

Lie on your back on the floor with your knees bent. Press your stomach in to the floor and place your fingers over mid-stomach area. Breathing out, lift your head and shoulders off the floor, keeping your eyes on the ceiling. Return to the beginning and breathe in.

Repeat 10 times, each time feeling the stomach muscles working through your fingers, and keeping your lower back firmly on the floor.

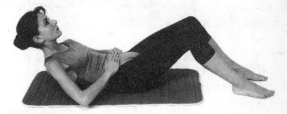

Bent leg raises

Lie on your stomach with your hands under your head. Keeping your upper body still, bend your left leg at the knee and raise it off the floor, feeling your bottom and lower back do the work.

Repeat 5 times working up to 20. Repeat on your other leg.

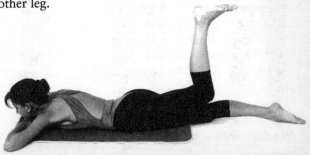

Hip flexor stretch

This also releases the lower back. Lie on your back with the correct pelvic alignment, your knees bent. Now straighten your left leg and bring the right leg into your body, clasping your hands round your right leg, just below the knee.

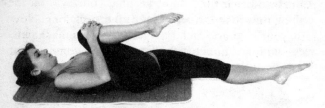

Bring the right leg in as far as you can, all the time concentrating on keeping the left leg straight on the floor. Hold the stretch just before the left leg does raise off the floor.

Hold for a count of 10. Repeat on the other side.

For Balance and Pelvic Strength

Ball of foot balance

Stand in correct pelvic position, feet an inch or two (2½–5 cm) apart. Now rise up on to the balls of your feet, keeping the centre of your body strong, and your shoulders back. Raise your arms toward the ceiling.

Concentrate on staying as solid and still as you can. Feel your bottom working. When you can maintain this

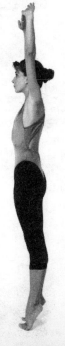

balance for a count of 10, move your heels up and down 10 times.

Kneeling arm and leg lifts

Kneel on all fours, keeping your hands and knees square. Flatten your back and pull in your stomach to maintain a pelvic tilt.

Look towards the floor to keep your neck long. Now raise your right arm and left leg off the floor, as shown, and hold for a count of 10. Repeat on the other side.

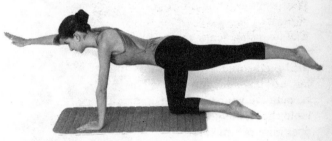

Groin and Hamstring Releases

Lying hamstring stretch

Lie on your back on the floor, your knees bent. Now bring your right leg in towards your chest, clasping your hands behind your calf. Pull gently until you feel the stretch along the back

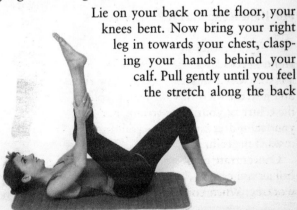

of your thigh. Breathe deeply as you stretch and try to relax.

Count to 10, and just before you come out of the stretch try to bring the thigh in a little further.

Repeat with the other leg.

Sitting hamstring stretch

Sit with your back straight, your left leg bent and your left foot flat on the floor. Your right leg should be out in front of you.

Now, using gentle pressure on the thigh just above the knee, straighten the right leg, making sure your foot is flexed with your toes pointing to the ceiling. Hold the position for a count of 10.

Repeat to the other side.

Sitting groin stretch

Sit on the floor with your legs bent and the soles of your feet together in front of you; back straight. Clasp ankles and gently rock your back forward until you feel a stretch inside the groin.

Concentrate on bringing the movement from

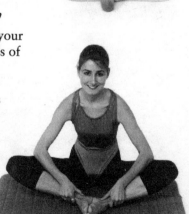

the lower back and don't slump. Hold the position for a count of 10. As your groin loosens, you can bring your feet nearer and nearer to your body.

Standing groin and hip flexor stretch

Stand sideways-on to the back of a sturdy chair, and hold it lightly for support throughout this exercise. Bring your right leg forward, with your knee bent as shown.

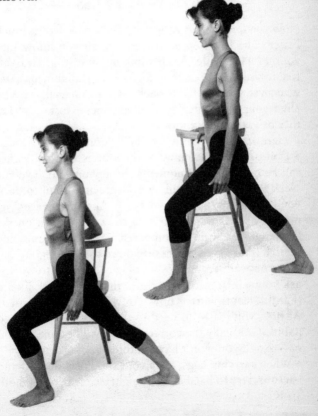

Take your left leg back on the ball of your foot, keeping your leg straight. Keep your body upright and in good pelvic alignment.

Now, move your right knee forward until you feel a stretch through your left hip, upper thigh and groin. Hold for a count of 10.

Repeat to the other side.

——BODY AWARENESS——

Now you understand your body and its mechanics much better. The last step is to translate all you know into your everyday life. Keep thinking slim, tall, straight. Keep thinking about that correct body alignment. And whenever you feel like slouching, remember that if you align yourself right, you look slimmer – instantly! Let that be your motivation.

Here are some pointers to help yourself all day long.

• Don't forget that many of the exercises and stretches can be done in odd moments throughout the day. The Neck Release and Shoulder Squeeze are useful to do if you have a desk job, for instance. And, in the evening, instead of sitting on your sofa to watch TV, sit on the floor and do a Sitting Groin Stretch or Sitting Hamstring Stretch (don't try stretches if you're cold, though).

• As you walk around – shopping or walking to work – ask yourself from time to time what you'd look like in that full-length mirror now. Are you correctly aligned? At first, you really do need to think about altering bad habits. Gradually the correct habits will become second nature and you won't have to think about them.

• When carrying bags, keep your shoulders relaxed and back, and try to balance the weight evenly between both arms.

• When reading, don't lean over the book; bring it up in front of you.

• When sitting in any kind of chair, make sure your bottom is well into the chair so that your spine is supported throughout its length by the back of the chair. If you sit with your bottom, say, halfway back, you will automatically end up in an ungainly position with a concertina middle, and an upper back forced into a slump. Sit like that all evening and you can see why you get bad body alignment!

• When driving, have the back of the seat as upright as you can and think about maintaining that sitting pelvic tilt as you drive. Your stomach won't bulge out under that seat belt, and this will also prevent the lower backache that plagues so many drivers.

Finally, remember you only have one body. If you treat it properly it will respond by looking good and feeling good well into old age. So give it the attention it deserves!

Chapter 6
NOW STAY SIZE 12 FOR EVER

So, now you're a trim, shapely size 12! We're going to make sure that you stay that way! Many people find weight and shape maintenance just as hard to achieve as getting there. You will be pleased to hear, then, that there is no truth in the much-discussed idea that once you've lost weight you have to exist on a low-calorie diet for the rest of your life in order to stay slim. You don't. What you do need to do, however, is to eat the right type of diet, and the right amount for you. If you follow all the advice in this chapter, you should be able to eat at least 2000 calories a day, and still keep that figure you've just worked so hard to attain.

And 2000 calories a day represents a little more than Britain's Department of Health's estimate of 1940 calories a day for an average nineteen- to forty-nine-year-old woman.

The keys to success with my system are as follows:

• Gradual adjustment to a higher intake of food after dieting.

• A maintenance diet high in carbohydrates and with other stay-slim food factors.

• Sensible food management: planning your diet to suit yourself, and to cope with day-to-day problems.

• An activity programme to keep that fat off you for good.

So let's take those four points and look at them in detail.

Gradual adjustment to a higher intake of food after dieting

Many people begin putting on weight again the very day they finish their slimming diet. And they don't stop until they've put back every ounce they so painstakingly lost.

Most of these women say that they finished the diet, weighed themselves a couple of days afterwards (having not binged in the meantime) and found to their horror that they'd put on 4 or 5 pounds. Having discovered this, they then felt so disheartened that they simply abandoned any idea of following a careful maintenance diet.

What people often don't realize is that a gain of a few pounds at the end of a strict diet, and when you start eating 'normally', is usual. It is not only usual, it is inevitable. The weight gain that worries so many women, what they see as a sign of their own failure, is called the 'glycogen gain', and it isn't fat. It's simply the body restoring its levels of liquid glucose and water. These levels, if you remember, caused you to lose a lot of weight quickly at the start of your diet.

When you drop the number of calories you consume to a level that causes you to lose weight, your glycogen stores deplete first and then the body starts burning up fat. When a normal calorie level is resumed, the glycogen stores then return very quickly.

This doesn't mean your diet hasn't worked, or that you are over-eating. And it is rare for the glycogen return to cause you to put on more than 3 or 4 pounds.

This glycogen gain is one reason why I find that the best way to come off a reduced-calorie diet is to step back up gradually to an intake of around 2000 calories a day. This is because the glycogen gain then happens much more slowly and is less noticeable, because you're still burning off fat during the week or so that you're building up to your final maintenance level.

The second advantage of a gradual return to eating more is psychological. It seems to stop people having the urge to throw the diet to the wind and grab the biscuits. You know, the 'Oh, good, the diet's finished, now I can reward myself' syndrome.

So when you have finished the 21-day schedule, you will find on pages 229–232 your programme for Days 22–28 – this transition period between weight-loss eating and maintenance eating. Don't skip it!

You should end up on the morning of Day 29 at approximately the same weight you were on Day 22.

In other words, although you've spent a week eating less than you will from now on (albeit more calories than you did throughout the 21-day diet), your actual weight has remained static because your glycogen stores have been gradually replacing themselves.

Now you are ready to move on to the maintenance diet itself.

A maintenance diet high in carbohydrates and with other stay-slim food factors

Eat plenty of bread and potatoes and pasta and rice, and you can stay slim for life! Carbohydrate foods – the ones that for so long were regarded as 'fattening' – are now known to be the ones our bodies prefer to use as fuel.

The glycogen stores in our bodies (see above) are the 'instant fuel' that we use for energy throughout the day, so the body is constantly replacing this glycogen to provide a ready source of energy when it's needed.

And the glycogen stores are produced, in the main, from the carbohydrate foods that we eat. Only about 10 per cent of the fat that we eat is used by the liver to make glycogen. That means that, unless we are indulging in fat burning aerobic exercise (see chart, page 169), the surplus fat is more likely to be converted to body fat.

However, if you eat a high carbohydrate diet, the body has to work much harder to convert surplus carbohydrate into fat. It *can* do it, but carbohydrate is not the body's prime choice for laying down fat. Protein *can't* be laid down as fat, so that only leaves fat.

The moral: Eat a high-carbohydrate diet that is also quite low in fat and you need never worry quite so much about calories again.

This was proved by the famous Cornell (USA) University research, where people who were allowed to eat as much carbohydrate as they liked, but had to restrict fats, actually lost weight while not, officially, dieting at all!

So why, then, do so many people who enjoy bread, potatoes, rice, pasta and other carbohydrate-rich foods, still stay fat? The answer, I am sure, lies in what they eat with and on their carbohydrates. Bread covered with lashings of butter, baked potatoes topped with even more butter, pasta topped with a double-cream sauce, rice fried instead of boiled: these are just some examples of how you can spoil a good carbohydrate food with a high-fat addition.

The secret is, when you're hungry, fill up on carbohydrates and don't ever feel guilty. But eat them with a reduced-fat accompaniment.

You also want to watch out for the hidden fat in foods that you may consider to be high carbohydrate. Croissants, for example, are approximately 20 per cent fat by weight; Victoria sponge cake is 26 per cent fat by weight.

And here I'd like to take a minute to explain the difference between *complex* carbohydrates and *simple* carbohydrates.

Complex carbohydrates are, in easy terms, natural, complete, unprocessed carbohydrates containing all their original fibre and usually plenty of vitamins and minerals, too. These are foods such as root vegetables, bananas, wholegrain rice, oats and pulses. Wholegrain breads and pasta are also complex carbohydrates, although they have been through a manufacturing process. Bread, of course, has a little added fat or oil (usually around 2 per cent by weight).

All fruits and vegetables are also complex carbohydrates although the World Health Organization lists them separately from the higher-calorie root vegetables, grains, pulses and nuts, probably because they have a high water content and are more useful for their antioxidant, vitamin and mineral content than for a significant source of carbohydrate energy.

And that is exactly why fruits and vegetables are so important on your weight maintenance plan. High on nutrients and low on calories and fat, they should be a very regular and important part of your diet.

Simple carbohydrates are, in easy terms, refined, processed, high-carbohydrate foods that have been stripped of all or most of their fibre and, often, of vitamins and minerals. Sugar is the prime example. It is a pure carbohydrate, but contains no fibre, no vitamins or minerals. It is highly refined and very quickly absorbed. Syrup and honey are other simple carbohydrates. Most confectionery consists of simple carbohydrates with colourings, flavourings, etc., and sometimes added fat.

For the purposes of staying slim, it is the complex carbohydrates that you should be eating more of in your diet. Think twice about the simple carbohydrates! This isn't because your body doesn't enjoy burning off the simple carbohydrates as energy just as much as it enjoys using the complex carbohydrates, but simple carbohydrates have a couple of disadvantages.

To begin with, they will not leave you feeling full for long, which is what the complex carbohydrates do. They are so quickly absorbed into your digestive system that you will feel hungry again too quickly after eating.

Secondly, if you eat too many simple carbohydrates at the expense of the complex ones, you may not get enough of the nutrients you need for good health.

Thirdly, simple carbos are often combined with fat in, for instance, chocolate, puddings, cakes and biscuits.

White bread, white rice and white pasta, by the way, are *not* simple carbohydrates. They are much more useful within your diet than, say, sugar. They all contain fibre and various vitamins and minerals and will keep you feeling full for longer than the simple carbohydrates will. But they *have* been stripped of some of their natural fibre by processing and are therefore not quite as good for your diet as their wholegrain counterparts.

So try to eat the whole varieties at least some, if not all, of the time. Remember, the less refined the product, the longer it will take your body to digest it, and the longer the hunger pangs will stay away.

The high-carbohydrate, reduced-fat way of eating is one you won't find a problem to adapt to; the 21-day diet itself has been getting you used to such a way of eating. On pages 233–239, you'll find a complete week's menus for your maintenance diet. The diet comprises approximately 2000 calories a day, and it is very similar in style to the 21-day diet. There is just more to eat, both in variety and quantity.

I suggest that on Days 29–35 you do follow this plan as closely as you can. It will get you used to what 2000 calories a day feels like, and it will build up your confidence in adding new foods to your diet.

The diet also incorporates one other very important principle in helping you to stay slim for life: the snacking principle. Your body metabolism works better – i.e., it burns up more food as fuel – if you eat frequently rather than (as so many people do) eating only one meal a day. Snacking can keep you slim!

And after Day 35

Once you've reached the end of the first week's maintenance diet, you can either repeat it for a further week if you don't feel confident yet, or you can now begin creating your own menus. You can do this with the help of the food charts at the end of the chapter. These will help you to identify what is, for instance, a high-carbohydrate, low-fat food, and what is a high-carbohydrate, high-fat food!

I don't intend or want you to spend the rest of your life counting calories or working out grams of fat in every last thing you eat; but, with a little common sense you will soon learn instinctively to get the balance of your diet right.

For your own interest – but please don't worry about working this out to the last percentage every day – you should be getting at least 50 per cent of your daily calories (energy) in the form of complex carbohydrate foods. You should be getting (if you want to stay slim) a maximum of 25 per cent of your daily calories in the form of fat (but 20 per cent is even better). Roughly 15 per cent of the daily calories should be in protein foods, and that leaves a *maximum* of 15 per cent for extras.

The extras are mainly simple carbohydrate foods like sugar and honey, and alcoholic drinks.

You should make sure you get at least two portions of fresh fruit a day, and at least three portions of fresh vegetables or salad.

An easy way to get the carbohydrate balance right is to think of the main part of each meal of the day as either bread, potatoes, rice, pasta, grains or pulses; then add a small amount of a high-protein, low-fat food, plus your fresh fruit and vegetables.

I also suggest giving yourself a daily fat allowance – of butter, oil or low-fat spread – of a maximum of, say, 200 calories.

This represents only 10 per cent (approximately) of your daily calories – although I have said you can have up to 25 per cent of your daily calories in fat – because fat is present in many of the other foods you will be eating, even when you choose low-fat foods. For example, reduced-fat Cheddar is 15 per cent fat by weight; chicken without skin is around 5 per cent fat by weight.

To help keep your fat levels low, on your maintenance diet you should continue using skimmed milk in your drinks, and use 'low-fat' alternatives whenever you can. For example, reduced-fat mayonnaise, very low-fat yogurt rather than whole yogurts, and oil-free French dressing, will all help the cause!

Here are a couple of examples of how this meal building works.

• You choose pasta as the main part of your meal, and you allow yourself a large portion. To it, you add a small portion of Bolognese sauce made from extra-lean mince and with oil from your allowance. You have a mixed side salad and a piece of fruit.

• You choose wholemeal French bread as the main part

of your meal, and you have a good, big slice. To it, you add a small portion of medium-fat soft cheese and you have some butter or low-fat spread from your daily fat allowance, to spread on your bread. You add some fresh tomato and onion salad, and a piece of fruit.

Work all your meals out like that and you really need never worry about your waistline again!

Don't forget: all the help you need with building the foundation of your high-carbohydrate, low-fat diet is contained in the food charts starting on page 240.

Sensible food management: planning your diet to suit yourself, and learning to cope with day-to-day problems

It is all very well theorizing about the kind of diet that will allow you to eat plenty, stay healthy and stay slim. But, I can hear you saying:

How does that translate into my own busy, individual lifestyle? How do I cope with my occasional urges for chocolate? How do I eat in restaurants or eat while I'm on the road?

The following are sensible, workable answers to those diet-breaking dilemmas that can affect us all.

• *Do I have to live without my favourite, but fattening, food?*

The simple answer to that is no. Even the most fanatical health-food freak always has at least one 'naughty food' skeleton in his cupboard. Mine are milk chocolate, Cornettos and wine; my husband's are toffee, chocolate biscuits and wine!

If the bulk of your diet is healthy – plenty of high-complex-carbohydrate, low-fat food – then I reckon you can safely allow yourself, say, 10 per cent of your daily calories for the more indulgent items like ice cream, cakes, chocolate, puddings, wine. Some of these foods will be higher in fat than others; for instance, wine contains no fat, while vanilla ice cream (dairy or non-dairy) is only about 8 per cent fat by weight, and milk chocolate is about 30 per cent fat.

So, if you consistently choose higher-fat items like chocolate, and indulge in 200 calories' worth (an average bar) every day, then it might be wise to cut your fat allowance down to 100 calories a day to compensate.

I've selected the most popular 'treat' foods, and on page 255 show you how much fat and how many calories they contain. This will help you select.

But what healthy, stay-slim eating is about, really, is *balance*. What people who stay slim do is use the 'swings and roundabouts' approach to food. If, one day, they eat two puddings and a packet of crisps, next day they won't have any treats.

We can look at the 7-day maintenance menu on pages 233–239 and see this principle working. Look at Day 29. You have a portion of chips with your main meal. First we've cut the fat in them because they're lower-fat oven chips; but, secondly, the rest of the day's food is very low in fat. For example, we've used only about 100 calories as a fat allowance, for spreading, etc. Our treat for the day is 2 glasses of wine, which is a no-fat item.

On Day 35, we have a roast-beef dinner followed by apple pie and cream. But we've cut fat, and calories, the rest of the day with a virtually fat-free lunch, and have used only 75 calories as a fat allowance (low-fat spread on the bread at breakfast and butter on the baked potato). And we've treated the apple pie and cream as this day's 'extra'.

• *I enjoy going out and entertaining. How do I fit my maintenance diet around that?*

As you've already seen, you can drink wine and eat well on the maintenance diet. These days, in the pub or wine bar, no one thinks you're boring if you have only one or two alcoholic drinks and choose a soft drink or mineral water in between. If you're going to eat in the pub, at most you can get wholemeal French bread, salad and ham. Cut any fat off the ham, leave most of any butter you're offered and you have a perfect high-carbohydrate meal!

If you eat nuts or crisps, you remember that they are high in fat, and you should balance the rest of your day's diet accordingly. I would also go without my daily 200-calorie 'treat' for the following day if I drank alcohol and ate snacks, too.

When entertaining at home *you* are in control and by now you should realize that you can cook tasty, interesting and filling meals that don't contain vast amounts of calories or fat. Look through your own recipe books and see if you can reduce the fat in your favourite recipes. I have found with most that you can at least halve the quantities of fat given in main-course dishes (for softening onions and other vegetables, browning meat and garnishing etc.) without affecting flavour or texture. Use the lowest-fat ingredients you can find (e.g., extra-lean mince, well-trimmed cutlets, and so on).

Low or fairly low-calorie starters are melon, vegetable soups made without cream, and marinated mushrooms. Fruit salad or fresh fruit always makes a refreshing dessert and you can hand round cream for those who want it.

If you're eating in restaurants or at other people's houses it usually isn't difficult to select wisely *if you want to*. I honestly think that most people who complain that they can't stay slim because they have to eat in restaurants a lot are people who eat out on a business account and don't like to turn down 'free' food!

Once you know a high-fat food from a low-fat food it shouldn't be hard to find your way through any menu, and to pick things that won't pile on pounds. If you're eating with friends you can always avoid adding butter to bread, ask for small portions of dessert and say no to second helpings.

The point is, do you eat out at a friend's home every night of the week? Every week, even? No? Remember that it isn't occasional indulgences that will make you fat, it is regular over-indulging in high-fat low-carbohydrate foods that will do so.

• *I'm very busy and I don't have much money. How do I find the time or money to eat well?*

Busy people who fit a lot into their lives generally have the knack of forward planning – and of eliminating unnecessary things from their lives. You can apply that to your diet, too. Planning what you are going to eat at home during the next few days, and doing one shop for that food, will save time in the long run. And it is just as quick and easy to eat low-fat high-carbohydrate food as it is to eat high-fat high-calorie food. What could be quicker or easier than a sandwich, or French bread and a low-fat cheese with tomatoes for lunch? Or a plate of quick-cook noodles with a jar of fresh tomato sauce for supper? What about a microwaved baked potato with a yogurt-based topping?

Fresh fruit is the quickest and easiest snack – or dessert – of all. Even breakfast can be as easy with a bowlful of wholegrain cereal and skimmed milk.

Most of the high-carbohydrate foods are also low on cost; bread, potatoes, rice, pasta and pulses are all just about the lowest-cost foods you can find.

• *I can be sensible about food most of the time, but now and then I binge. How can I stop this happening?*

Women seem to binge more than men do, and I am sure it is because of their hormonal 'ups and downs'. Most women tend to binge in the few days before their menstrual cycle starts. This can be controlled by regular snacking on high complex carbohydrate foods during those danger days. The worst thing you can do if you have a binge tendency is to go for hours without eating anything. Eat regular snacks, such as a small slice of wholemeal bread with a little low-fat cheese; rye crispbreads with a hard-boiled egg; a banana; some dried fruit or an apple. Feeding your system with these high-carbohydrate snacks keeps your blood sugar at a constant, steady level and will prevent the urge to binge.

Generally speaking, the healthier your everyday diet, the less often the urge to binge will arrive. Another tip is to save your day's treat – for example, a 200-calorie chocolate bar or an ice cream – to follow your main meal or your lunch. Sugary items eaten when you are hungry tend to make you crave more sugary items.

• *Sometimes I get so hungry I've just got to eat something, even though it isn't mealtime. What should I do?*

Eat something. If you have genuine hunger pangs you shouldn't feel guilty about eating. Perhaps you've been using up more energy than usual. You can either bring your next meal forward, if that's convenient, or add a snack to your day's eating – a high-carbohydrate snack, of course.

It is also sensible to pay attention to your own 'body clock', and plan your day's meals around that. For instance, I always feel ravenous around 5.30 p.m. – and I've now learnt to allow for some bread, a banana or something about then (I'm too busy to eat a full meal at that time). Someone else I know becomes very bad-tempered if she doesn't get a good substantial breakfast; so, of course, now she eats a big breakfast, has a medium-sized lunch and a light meal in the evening.

Everyone has his or her own particular 'hungry time of day'. Discover yours and allow for it.

Lastly, on hunger: don't mistake greed for hunger. When you're hungry, you eat your main meal and feel full. Then someone brings round a dessert trolley and suddenly you can manage a huge slice of gâteau! That is not hunger making you eat that dessert. Be aware of the difference, and it'll be easy to decide what you actually need.

You can maintain your new weight and never feel hungry again; but you may, sometimes, be caught out by foods that tempt you to eat more stay you meant to.

An activity programme to keep that fat off you for good

Once you are the shape you want to be, it may be tempting to stop your activity programme and take a rest. On the other hand, you may find you have enjoyed the programme so much that you want to continue at the same level.

The first alternative is definitely not a good idea, and the second isn't completely necessary.

Why? If you stop exercising, the sad truth is that within months your body will have returned to its former, unfit, out-of-shape condition. Muscles need regular work to stay toned and strong; joints need regular use to stay supple; heart and lungs need work to keep fit. Also, if you stop exercising, you will find it harder to maintain your weight loss.

But, unless you want to enter body-building competitions, or perhaps become a top athlete or gymnast, neither is it necessary for you to work out for hours every day for the rest of your life. To maintain a good shape and a reasonable level of fitness, you want to maintain a programme that is somewhere between the two extremes.

The following outlines the Maintenance Activity Programme that will keep you looking and feeling great.

——THE MAINTENANCE ACTIVITY—— PROGRAMME

Body Contouring

Do the body contouring super programme three times a week on alternate days. One set should be enough, but once a week or so do two sets just for fun.

Spot Reducing

Once you're the shape you want to be, you can dispense with any of the spot reducing routines that you have been doing. If you feel your problem areas beginning to bother you again, try twice-weekly sets of your regular exercises until you feel comfortable again.

Fat Burning

A regular fat burning programme will help you to avoid putting on weight again. And it will keep you fit for everyday life. So, do a walk – or an aerobic alternative – at least three times a week. You needn't be too concerned about the length of time you are out walking, as long as you achieve a brisk, low-intensity aerobic pace for at least 20 minutes of your walk. Remember, anything over 20 minutes and you're burning more and more fat. If you've always had trouble maintaining your weight loss in the past, it might pay you to walk for longer.

Here is a specimen programme for the average person; adapt it to suit yourself.

Walk three times a week on alternate days to the body-contouring programme.

Day 1

45 minutes *walk*, the middle 30 minutes *brisk*.
• Aim to cover: 3 miles.

Day 2

30 minutes *walk*, the middle 20 minutes *brisk*.
• Aim to cover: 2 miles.

Day 3

1 hour *walk*, the middle 30 minutes *brisk*.
• Aim to cover: 4 miles.

For extra fat burning – and variety – don't forget the potential of various other activities, such as swimming and cycling. Everyone needs a change, so don't be frightened to try something different.

Body Awareness

Once you've reached your target shape, it's vital that you don't slip back into old, bad posture habits, or forget all you learnt in Chapter 5. All day, every day, you should remember how to stand and how to sit. Think about your body alignment whatever you do.

And, remember to build little exercises into your daily life to help keep yourself supple and firm. Try bottom squeezes while you're sitting at a desk, or shoulder or neck releases while you're washing-up.

Bodies are meant to be used, so use yours!

And lastly …

Before I leave you with the maintenance diets and food charts, I want to say that I hope you feel pleased with yourself and as delighted as I do that you've finally reached your target size. I know how much it must mean to you – and how much it will continue to do so.

But eating the right foods and exercising your body properly in the long term has other advantages than just being able to fit into that longed-for dress. Feeling healthy, full of self-confidence, optimism and energy are the most frequent benefits newly-slim people tell me they experience. Hopefully, you began to feel this way from Day 1 of the diet and you can continue to do so in the years ahead, so long as you stay with my simple 'Size 12' eating and activity philosophy.

Why not make a list now of all the good things you've experienced since you decided to shape up with this 'Size 12' programme? Write down everything – apart from your shape itself – that makes you so glad you achieved your goal. For instance, your list might include any of the following:

• Better skin
• More self-confidence
• Waking up with a sense of anticipation rather than depression
• Improved general health

228

- Better digestion
- Increased energy
- Fewer aches and pains
- Reduced PMT
- Easier periods
- No more binges
- Stronger and fitter body
- Healthier gums, hair and nails
- More compliments
- More attention from people in general
- More enjoyable social life
- Improved sex life
- More able to cope with everyday problems
- Chores become less of an effort

I'm sure you will have plenty of your own feelings and comments to add! And, if at any time in the future there are days when you have even a faint inclination to abandon your body to its own fate again, take out that list and read through it a couple of times.

Always remember that you owe it to yourself to find the time to look after your body. Now – and for the rest of your life.

——THE TRANSITION—— PROGRAMME

Start on this plan as soon as you have finished the 21-day diet.

<u>DAYS 22–26 inclusive</u>

For the first five days you will be eating approximately 1250 calories a day. To achieve this, all you have to do is to return to Days 3–7 of the 21-day diet (see pages 30–45) and follow those days, which are based on 1100 calories a day, but adding one of the following to your daily diet. Each item contains approximately 150 calories.

• 50 g (2 oz) wholemeal bread with a very little low-fat spread
• 175 g (6 oz) potato, baked, boiled or instant mashed
• 25 g (1 oz) no-added-sugar muesli, plus 15 g (1/2 oz) dried fruit of your choice
• 140 g (5 oz) (boiled weight) rice or pasta
• 1 tub of diet yogurt and 1 large banana
• 1 average wholemeal roll with a very little low-fat spread and 1 teaspoon low-sugar jam, or 2 teaspoons pure fruit spread
• 25 g (1 oz) shelled unsalted almonds or hazelnuts

Vary your 'extra' choice as much as possible. Eat it whenever you like – either as a snack, dessert, or to increase the portion size of any meal.

DAYS 27 and 28

For the last two days of your week's transition, you will be eating approximately 1500 calories a day. To manage this, just follow the two days' diets, as laid out below, and add one of the following to each day. Each item contains approximately 100 calories; just choose whichever you like, and eat or drink it as instructed.

• 1 x 140 ml (5 fl oz, 1/4 pint) glass of dry or medium-dry white wine, to be drunk with your evening meal
• 50 g (2 oz) vanilla ice cream as a dessert for lunch or your evening meal
• One chewy or crunchy muesli or granola bar, to be eaten in addition to your mid-morning or afternoon snack, or as a dessert for lunch or your main meal

• 25 g (1 oz) slice wholemeal bread with a very little low-fat spread and 1 teaspoon low-sugar jam or 2 teaspoons pure fruit spread, to be eaten as a mid-morning or afternoon snack or added to breakfast
• 2 dark rye or oatbran Ryvitas, topped with 1 triangle of cheese spread or 25 g (1 oz) half-fat soft cheese added to your mid-morning or afternoon snack

On both days you have an allowance of 275 ml (10 fl oz, 1/2 pint) skimmed milk and items from the Unlimiteds list (see page 17).

Day 27

Breakfast
• 50 g (2 oz) no-added-sugar muesli, with 140 ml (5 fl oz, 1/4 pint) skimmed milk *extra* to allowance
• 1 fruit choice* (see page 18)

Mid-morning
• 1 large banana

Lunch
• 75 g (3 oz) slice wholemeal baguette plus 50 g (2 oz) extra-lean ham, a little low-fat spread to cover bread, a large mixed salad of choice and mustard to taste
• 1 diet fruit yogurt, any flavour

Mid-afternoon
• 25 g (1 oz) dried apricots, peaches, sultanas or raisins

Evening
• 75 g (3 oz) (dry weight) spaghetti, boiled and topped with half a jar of chilled tomato sauce plus 2 table-spoons grated Parmesan cheese and served with a green salad

231

Day 28

Breakfast
• 25 g (1 oz) branflakes or Puffed Wheat, with 110 ml (4 fl oz) skimmed milk *extra* to allowance
• 25 g (1 oz) slice wholemeal toast with a little low-fat spread and 1 teaspoon low-sugar jam or 2 teaspoons pure fruit spread
• 1 fruit choice* (see page 18)

Mid-morning
• 1 large banana

Lunch
• Sandwich of 2 slices of wholemeal bread from a large, medium-cut loaf with a little low-fat spread and filled with 40 g (1½ oz) reduced-fat Cheddar-style cheese, with sliced tomato
• 1 x 300 g (12 oz) can lentil soup
• 1 satsuma or kiwifruit

Mid-afternoon
• 1 diet fruit yogurt, any flavour

Evening
•110 g (4 oz) roast or grilled chicken with skin removed; 1 x 250 g (9 oz) baked potato topped with 1 tablespoon natural fromage frais; 110 g (4 oz) peas; 1 tablespoon stuffing of choice; fat-skimmed gravy

*From Day 27 onwards, you can add the following to your C-rich fruit choice: 1 x 140 ml (5 fl oz, ¼ pint) glass of unsweetened orange or grapefruit or mixed citrus fruit juice.

And you can add the following to your fruit choice: 1 x 140 ml (5 fl oz, ¼ pint) glass of unsweetened apple, pineapple, tomato or grape juice.

However, you should not choose more than one fruit juice serving a day. The rest of your fruit choices should be whole fruit. Whole fruit contains fibre which will help to fill you up much better than the juice alone.

——THE MAINTENANCE DIET——

DAYS 29–35

Weigh yourself today

You should weigh approximately the same as you did this time last week. Now you're ready to begin maintenance eating.

The plan below is approximately 2000 calories a day. This should be about right for the majority of women following the maintenance activity programme; however, people do vary in what they can eat. You may find (especially if you're tall and/or relatively young) that you can eat more and not put on weight. If, on the other hand, you're quite small and/or are over fifty, you may find that you have to eat a little less to maintain your weight. As the weeks progress you will discover your own level and adjust your intake accordingly.

Each day you follow the basic diet, and *add one of the following to your daily diet*. Each item contains approximately 200 calories.

• 2 x 140 ml (5 fl oz, 1/4 pint) glasses dry or medium white wine
• 75 g (3 oz) ice cream, or choc ice, with a wafer
• 1 x 140 ml (5 fl oz, 1/4 pint) glass wine, plus 50 g (2 oz) of ice cream
• 50 g (2 oz) slice of fruit cake
• 1 wholemeal fruit scone plus 2 teaspoons low-sugar jam
• 1 large wholemeal bap with a little low-fat spread, plus 2 teaspoons honey or 15 g (1/2 oz) reduced-fat Cheddar-style cheese
• Extra 50 g (2 oz) (dry weight) pasta or rice, boiled

Daily allowances: 275 ml (10 fl oz, ¹/2 pint) skimmed milk.

Unlimiteds: See page 17.

Day 29

Breakfast
• 1 medium (size 3) boiled egg; 2 slices bread or toast from a large wholemeal medium-cut loaf, plus a little low-fat spread to cover and 2 teaspoons low-sugar marmalade or jam
• 1 C-rich fruit choice (see page 18)

Mid-morning
• 1 x 40 g (1¹/2 oz) all-fruit bar

Lunch
• 2 thin slices (40 g, 1¹/2 oz) corned beef with 2 slices wholemeal bread from a large medium-cut loaf; plus large mixed salad
• 1 x 125 g (4¹/2 oz) tub low-fat natural yogurt, with 2 teaspoons honey, plus 15 g (¹/2 oz) sultanas

Mid-afternoon
• 1 banana and 1 apple

Evening
• 1 average (225 g, 8 oz) trout, baked or grilled, served with 140 g (5 oz) oven chips, baked or grilled, and 110 g (4 oz) peas

Day 30

Breakfast
• 70 g (2¹/2 oz) muesli with 140 ml (5 fl oz, ¹/4 pint) skimmed milk *extra* to allowance
• 1 C-rich fruit choice (see page 18)

Mid-morning
• 1 large banana

Lunch
• 1 wholemeal pitta bread with 110 g (4 oz) hummus, plus a selection of chopped salad items such as tomato, pepper, radish, onion and crisp lettuce
• 1 fruit choice (see page 18)

Mid-afternoon
• 1 x 25 g (1 oz) slice wholemeal bread with 25 g (1 oz) Edam or reduced-fat Cheddar

Evening
• Mushroom risotto: Sauté 110 g (4 oz) sliced mushrooms in 1 tablespoon of oil, stirring. Add 110 g (4 oz) dry weight risotto rice (*arborio*) and stir to coat. Add vegetable stock to cover and simmer, adding extra stock as necessary, until rice is cooked. Add seasonings, 25 g (1 oz) peas or sweetcorn, simmer again and serve.

Day 31

Breakfast
• 1 x 225 g (8 oz) tub Greek sheep's milk yogurt
• 1 C-rich fruit choice (see page 18)
• 1 fruit choice (see page 18)

Mid-morning
• 1 x 40g (½ oz) all-fruit bar

Lunch
• 1 x 300 g (12 oz) can mixed vegetable soup
• Sandwich of 2 slices wholemeal bread from large medium-cut loaf, with 1 tablespoon peanut butter plus salad
• 1 satsuma

Mid-afternoon
• 1 diet fromage frais, any flavour

Evening
• Liver and noodle stir-fry: Cook 75 g (3 oz) noodles as instructed on the packet and drain. Stir-fry 110 g (4 oz) sliced lamb's liver in 1 dessertspoon corn oil with 1 extra-lean back bacon rasher, chopped. Add some chopped green pepper, tomato purée, stock and 1 dessertspoon paprika, simmer for a few minutes and toss with noodles to reheat.

Day 32

Breakfast
• As Day 30 (see page 234)

Mid-morning
• 1 large banana

Lunch
• 75 g (3 oz) wholemeal baguette with 25 g (1 oz) Stilton, plus 1 dessertspoon pickle and a little low-fat spread with large mixed salad
• 1 satsuma

Mid-afternoon
• 1 diet fromage frais, any flavour

Evening
• Chicken tandoori or tikka: Skin one medium chicken breast and cut in two. Mix 1 tablespoon tikka or tandoori paste with 3 tablespoons low-fat natural yogurt, and coat chicken. Leave to marinate, then bake for 45 minutes. Serve with 75 g (3 oz) (dry weight) rice plus a salad of tomato and onion, and one of chopped cucumber in natural yogurt.

Day 33

Breakfast
- 2 Weetabix with 140 ml (5 fl oz, 1/4 pint) skimmed milk *extra* to allowance
- 1 slice wholemeal bread from large medium-cut loaf, with low-fat spread and low-sugar marmalade

Mid-morning
- 1 C-rich fruit choice (see page 18)

Lunch
- 1 small tub diet coleslaw; 50 g (2 oz) luncheon tongue; 60 g (2 1/2 oz) French bread; 2 baby beetroots; tomato and lettuce salad
- 1 fruit choice

Mid-afternoon
- 25 g (1 oz) shelled hazelnuts
- 1 diet yogurt, any flavour

Evening
- 110 g (4 oz) (dry weight) spaghetti boiled and topped with half a jar (approximately 50 g, 2 oz) pesto, plus 1 tablespoon grated Parmesan cheese; green salad

Day 34

Breakfast
- 25 g (1 oz) branflakes with 75 ml (3 fl oz) skimmed milk

Mid-morning
- 1 fruit bar

Lunch
- 1 medium (size 3) hard-boiled egg with 1 level dessertspoon reduced-calorie mayonnaise

• 1 average wholemeal roll with a little low-fat spread; salad of tomatoes and onion with a little olive oil dribbled on
• 1 large banana

Mid-afternoon
• 1 fruit choice (see page 18)

Evening
• 225 g (8 oz) white fish fillet of choice, poached or microwaved and topped with 140 ml (5 fl oz, 1/4 pint) cheese sauce made from skimmed milk and 25 g (1 oz) reduced-fat grated Cheddar-style cheese (make the roux using 1 g [1/4 oz] low-fat spread and 1 heaped teaspoon flour). Serve with 225 g (8 oz) boiled potatoes, 50 g (2 oz) peas and 110 g (4 oz) broccoli.
• 1 diet fromage frais, any flavour

Day 35

Breakfast
• As Day 5 (see page 37)

Mid-morning
• 1 C-rich fruit choice (see page 18)

Lunch
• 75 g (3 oz) wholemeal baguette plus 1 small tub natural cottage cheese; mixed salad and 1 x 125 g (4 1/2 oz) tub diet coleslaw

Mid-afternoon
• 1 fruit choice (see page 18)

Evening
• 110 g (4 oz) lean roast beef; 1 x 275 g (10 oz) baked potato; 110 g (4 oz) cabbage; 110 (4 oz) carrots; fat-

skimmed gravy and 1 teaspoon horseradish; 7 g
(¹/4 oz) butter for potato
• 1 average serving single crust apple pie plus an
average serving of aerosol cream

DAY 35 Onwards

You may repeat this week, if you like. Remember: when
you feel confident to plan your own diet, use the food
charts on pages 240–256 to help you choose a balanced
diet.

Chapter 7
YOUR GUIDE TO CALORIES AND FAT

——HIGH-CARBOHYDRATE,——
LOW-FAT FOODS

The foods in this chart are those that should form the core of your diet. They are high complex carbohydrate foods which are also low, or relatively low, in fat.

Fat is given as a percentage of the total *weight* of the food, rather than as a percentage of the total calories.

• = trace of fat
= no fat

	Calories	Per cent of fat content by weight
Breads and Crispbreads		
All are per 25 g (1 oz) unless otherwise stated.		
Bread		
Brown	60	2.2
Wheatgerm; e.g., Hovis	61	2.2
White	63	1.7
Wholemeal	59	2.7
Wholemeal, per slice from a large, medium-cut loaf	75	2.7
Pitta bread, white, 1 (70 g, 2½ oz)	180	1.2
Pitta bread, brown, 1 (70 g, 2½ oz)	165	1.2
Pitta, mini, 1	90	1.2
French bread, white	85	2.0
French bread, brown	75	1.5

	Calories	Per cent of fat content by weight
Bap, wholemeal	125	2.2
Petit Pain, granary, 1	105	2.0
Crispbread		
Ryvita, 1	25	2.1

Breakfast Cereals
All are per 25 g (1 oz) unless otherwise stated.

	Calories	Per cent of fat content by weight
All Bran	75	5.0
Branflakes	90	0.5
Cornflakes	100	1.6
Muesli, no added sugar	105	7.5
Porridge oats, raw	110	8.7
Porridge, made up with water, per 100 ml (3½ fl oz)	45	0.9
Shredded Wheat, 1	80	3.0
Weetabix, 1	65	3.4

Dried Fruits
All are per 25 g (1 oz) unless otherwise stated.
   All have only a trace of fat.

	Calories	
Apricots	45	•
Currants	60	•
Dates, stoned	70	•
Dates, each	15	•
Figs	53	•
Figs, each	30	•
Peaches	53	•
Prunes, stoned	46	•
Prunes, each	10	•
Raisins	61	•
Sultanas	62	•

	Calories	Per cent of fat content by weight

Grains

All are dry weight per 25 g (1 oz) unless otherwise stated.

	Calories	Per cent of fat content by weight
Couscous	94	1.0
Flour, white	87	1.2
Flour, wholemeal	80	2.0
Pasta, all shapes, white	105	1.0
Pasta, all shapes, brown	95	1.0
Pasta, white, boiled	30	0.3
Pasta, brown, boiled	30	0.9
Pearl barley	90	1.7
Rice, white	100	0.5
Rice, brown	95	1.0
Rice, white, boiled	32	0.3
Rice, brown, boiled	30	0.5
Semolina	87	1.8

Pulses

Pulses are virtually the perfect food. They are not only very high in carbohydrates and low in fat, but they also contain up to 20 per cent protein by weight. Eat pulses regularly.

All are dry weight per 25 g (1 oz) unless otherwise stated.

	Calories	Per cent of fat content by weight
Baked beans in tomato sauce, canned	16	0.5
Butter beans	68	1.1
Butter beans, boiled or canned	23	0.3
Chick peas	80	5.7
Chick peas, boiled or canned	36	3.3
Haricot beans	67	1.6
Kidney beans	68	1.7
Kidney beans, boiled or canned	25	0.5
Lentils, brown or green	76	1.0
Lentils, brown or green, boiled	25	0.5

	Calories	Per cent of fat content by weight
Lentils, red	85	1.5
Lentils, red, boiled	25	0.5
Lentil soup, per 100 ml (3½ fl oz)	99	3.7
Split peas	77	1.0
Split peas, boiled	30	0.3

Nuts

Most nuts are listed under *Low-Carbohydrate, High-Fat Foods.*

Chestnuts, shelled, per 25 g (1 oz)	42	2.7

Vegetables

The vegetables listed here have a higher carbohydrate – and calorie – content than the vegetables listed on pages 250–1. They also contain reasonable amounts of protein.

All are per 25 g (1 oz) unless otherwise stated.

Avocado, half a medium	200	4.5
Corn-on-the-cob, 1 medium	80	2.0
Peas, fresh, shelled or frozen	41	0.4
Potatoes:		
Boiled	80	0.1
Mashed with 10 g (½ oz)		
low-fat spread	116	4.0
Instant mashed	90	0.5
Baked, average 225 g (8 oz) potato	236	0.1
Roast, large chunks	150	4.5
(For chips and crisps, see *Treats* list		
on page 255.)		
Sweet potato	85	0.6
Sweetcorn kernels	76	2.0
Sweetcorn, whole baby cobs	25	0.5

——HIGH-PROTEIN, LOW-FAT——
FOODS

The foods listed here contain little or no carbohydrates, so always eat them with a high-carbohydrate food as part of a main meal.

For the purposes of this section, 'low fat' means 5 per cent fat or less. All are per 100 g (3½ oz) or 100 ml (3½ fl oz), unless otherwise stated.

	Calories	Per cent of fat content by weight
Cheese		
Cottage cheese, standard	96	4.0
Cottage cheese, diet	71	0.4
Quark low-fat	125	1.0
Fish		
Cod fillet	76	0.7
Coley fillet	73	0.6
Haddock fillet	73	0.6
Halibut steak	92	2.4
Monkfish fillet	73	0.6
Plaice fillet	91	2.2
Salmon, smoked	142	4.5
Trout, rainbow fillet	135	4.0
Tuna steak, fresh	157	4.5
Tuna in brine, drained	87	0.6
Haddock, smoked, fillet	100	1.0
Seafood		
Crabmeat	127	5.0
Prawns, shelled	107	1.8
Mussels, shelled	87	2.0
Scallops, shelled	105	1.4
Squid	71	0.8

	Calories	Per cent of fat content by weight
Meat and Poultry		
Chicken, meat only (no skin or bone)	120	5.0
Duck, raw weight, meat only (no skin)	122	4.8
Beef, topside	156	4.4
Kidneys, lamb's	90	2.7
Ham, extra-lean	120	5.0
Rabbit, meat only	124	4.0
Turkey, light meat	103	1.1
Turkey, dark meat	114	3.6
Veal	110	2.7
Vegetarian Foods		
Quorn	80	2.9
Tofu	70	4.0
Yogurts and Fromage Frais		
Fromage frais, natural, low-fat	53	0.2
Yogurt, natural, low-fat	52	1.0
Yogurt, fruit, low-fat	95	1.0

——HIGH-PROTEIN, MEDIUM-FAT—— FOODS

The foods listed here are good sources of protein, but contain between 5 and 15 per cent fat so you should choose them less often than the high-protein, low-fat foods listed previously.

All are per 100 g (3½ oz) or 100 ml (3½ fl oz) unless otherwise stated.

	Calories	Per cent of fat content by weight
Cheese		
Cheddar, reduced-fat style	285	15.0
Low-fat soft cheese, e.g., Shape	133	8.5
Fish		
Fish fingers, grilled	178	7.5
Fish, frozen battered portion, fried in oil	200	10.0
Herring, grilled	199	13.0
Kipper, grilled	200	12.0
Pilchards in tomato sauce	126	5.4
Salmon, fresh, fillet	182	12.0
Tuna canned in oil, drained	122	5.0
Eggs		
Size 2 egg, each	90	11.0
Size 3 egg, each	80	11.0
Size 4 egg, each	75	11.0
Egg, scrambled with 7 g (¼ oz) low-fat spread and dash (100 ml, 3½ fl oz) skimmed milk	185	14.0

	Calories	*Per cent of fat content by weight*
Meat and Poultry		
Chicken, roast, meat and skin	216	14.0
Beef, extra-lean, minced	190–210	7.0–10.0
Beefburger, low-fat, grilled	150	7.0
Beef, roast, lean only	190	9.0
Beef steak, rump, lean only, grilled	190	7.5
Corned beef	217	12.0
Duck, roast, lean only	190	9.0
Lamb, leg, roast, lean only	190	8.0
Lamb, chop, well-trimmed, weighed with bone	133	12.0
Liver, lamb's	180	10.0
Pork, roast, lean only	185	7.0
Pork fillet	185	7.0
Sausages, low-fat, grilled	180	8.0
Venison, meat only	198	6.0
Yogurt and Fromage Frais		
Fromage frais, natural	114	8.0
Yogurt, Greek ewe's	90	7.5

——FRESH FRUITS AND JUICES——

None of these foods contains more than a trace of fat or protein; they are virtually pure carbohydrate foods and low (or lowish) in calories because of their high water content. Fruit generally contains plenty of vitamin C, minerals and fibre, so eat at least two portions a day. Fruit canned in natural juice and drained will have a similar calorie count but not as much vitamin C or fibre, so fresh is preferable.

	Calories	Per cent of fat content by weight
Fruit		
All are per item unless otherwise stated.		
All are very low in fat.		
Apple, dessert	50	•
Apple, cooking, per 25 g (1 oz)	10	•
Apricot, fresh	15	•
Banana, 1 small	60	•
1 medium	80	•
1 large	100	•
Blackberries, per 25 g (1 oz)	10	•
Blackcurrants, per 25 g (1 oz)	10	•
Cherries, per 25 g (1 oz)	10	•
Damsons, with stones, per 25 g (1 oz)	10	•
Date, fresh	15	•
Fig, fresh	30	•
Gooseberries, dessert, per 25 g (1 oz)	10	•
Gooseberries, cooking, per 25 g (1 oz)	5	•
Grapefruit, half	20	•
Grapes, per 25 g (1 oz)	15	•
Kiwifruit	30	•
Lemon, 1 whole	20	•

	Calories	Per cent of fat content by weight
Lime	15	•
Mango	100	•
Melon, 200 g (7 oz) slice	25	•
Nectarine	50	•
Orange	50	•
Peach	50	•
Pear, average	50	•
large	70	•
Pineapple, 1-ring slice	25	•
Plum, dessert	20	•
Raspberries, per 25 g (1 oz)	7	•
Rhubarb, 1 large stick	10	•
Satsuma or tangerine	20	•
Strawberries, per 25 g (1 oz)	7	•

Juices

Fresh juice is better than long life; fresh fruit contains fibre, juice contains very little. Fruit will therefore keep you feeling full for longer than juice, so it is preferable to choose whole fruit rather than juice most of the time.

All are per 25 ml (1 fl oz), unless otherwise stated. An average glass equals 125 ml (4½ fl oz, ¼ pint)

Apple	10	•
Grape	15	•
Grapefruit	10	•
Mixed citrus	10	•
Mixed vegetable	5	•
Orange	10	•
Pineapple	11	•
Tomato	5	•

——FRESH VEGETABLES——

None of these vegetables contain more than a trace of fat. They contain a little protein, but their calories are mostly complex carbohydrate. The calorie counts are low because vegetables have a high water content. The vitamin, fibre and mineral content of these vegetables are excellent, and they have enormous filling power. Eat fresh vegetables or salad with *every* meal.

Frozen vegetables have a similar calorie count and can be used as a substitute for fresh; the freezing process allows almost all the nutrients to be retained. Keep canned vegetables for occasional use only.

All calories are per 25 g (1 oz) unless otherwise stated. All are very low in fat.

	Calories	Per cent of fat content by weight
Artichoke, globe	10	•
Artichoke, Jerusalem	5	•
Asparagus, 1 spear	5	•
Aubergine	4	•
Beans, broad	15	•
Beans, French	10	•
Beans, runner	5	•
Beansprouts	5	•
Beetroot	12	•
Broccoli	5	•
Brussels sprouts	5	•
Cabbage, all kinds	4	•
Carrots	5	•
Cauliflower	4	•
Celeriac	4	•
Celery, 1 stick	3	•

	Calories	Per cent of fat content by weight
Chicory	3	•
Chinese leaves	3	•
Courgettes	4	•
Cucumber	3	•
Leek	5	•
Lettuce, all kinds	3	•
Marrow	3	•
Mushrooms	5	•
Mustard and cress, whole box	5	•
Onion	10	•
Onion, spring, 1	3	•
Parsnip	15	•
Pepper, green	4	•
other colours	8	•
Radish	3	•
Spinach	7	•
Swede	5	•
Tomato	4	•
1 average	10	•
Turnip	5	•
Watercress	5	•

For other vegetables, e.g., potatoes, see *High-Carbohydrate, Low-Fat Foods* on page 240.

——LOW-CARBOHYDRATE,——
HIGH-FAT FOODS

Because of their very high fat content, all the foods below should be eaten either in very small portions or just occasionally. Some contain good amounts of protein, but for protein intake it is better to choose from the high-protein, low- or medium-fat listings.

	Calories	Per cent of fat content by weight
Cheeses		
All are per 25 g (1 oz) unless otherwise stated.		
Brie	75	27.0
Camembert	75	23.0
Cheddar	101	33.5
Cheese spread	71	23.0
Cream cheese, full-fat	110	47.0
Danish Blue	89	29.0
Edam	76	23.0
Mozzarella, Italian	62	19.0
Eggs		
Egg, fried, 1 size 3	120	19.0
Cream		
All are per 100 ml (3½ fl oz) unless otherwise stated.		
Single	212	21.0
Whipping	332	35.0
Double	447	48.0

252

	Calories	Per cent of fat content by weight

Fats and Oils
All are per 25 g (1 oz) or 25 ml (1 fl oz)
unless otherwise stated.

	Calories	Per cent of fat content by weight
Butter	185	82.0
Low-fat spread	91	40.0
Very low-fat spread	57	25.0
Margarine, all types including sunflower	182	81.0
Oils, all kinds, e.g., corn, olive, vegetable	225	99.9

Fish
All are per 100 g (3½ oz) unless otherwise stated.

	Calories	Per cent of fat content by weight
Homemade or chip shop, batter-coated and fried	300	20.0
Scampi, battered and fried	316	17.5
Whitebait, deep-fried	525	47.5

Meat
All are per 100 g (3½ oz) unless otherwise stated.

	Calories	Per cent of fat content by weight
Beef, average minced	230	16.0
Bacon, back, average, grilled	405	33.0
Bacon, back, trimmed, grilled	290	17.0
Bacon, streaky, grilled	422	36.0
Lamb, shoulder, roast	316	26.0
Lamb, chops (including fat)	355	29.0
Duck, roast (including skin)	340	30.0
Liver sausage	310	27.0
Luncheon meat	310	27.0
Salami	490	45.0

	Calories	Per cent of fat content by weight
Sausages:		
Beef, grilled	265	17.0
Pork, grilled	318	25.0
Frankfurters	275	25.0
Tongue	213	16.0

Nuts
All are shelled weight per 100 g (3½ oz).

Almonds	565	53.5
Brazils	619	61.5
Hazelnuts	380	36.0
Peanuts, fresh or roasted and salted	570	49.0
Peanut butter	623	53.0
Walnuts	525	51.5

Pastry items
All are per 100 g (3½ oz).

Pastry, shortcrust	527	32.0
Pastry, flaky	565	40.0
Pork pie	376	27.0
Pastie, Cornish	330	20.0

Dressings
All are per 15 ml (1 tablespoon).

French dressing	98	70.0
Mayonnaise	108	78.0
Mayonnaise, reduced-calorie	45	28.0
Salad cream	45	27.0

——BAKERY ITEMS, SWEETS——
AND SNACKS

Many of the foods in this list are high in carbohydrates; however, they are usually rich in the 'not-so-good', simple carbohydrates. These foods frequently contain a great deal of fat, and are low in nutrients.

Like the low-carbohydrate, high-fat foods, the following should be eaten in small portions or just occasionally.

	Calories	Per cent of fat content by weight
Biscuits, digestive, each	75	20.0
Biscuits, chocolate, each	95	27.0
Cake, fruit, 50 g (2 oz) slice	165	11.0
Cake, Victoria sponge, 50 g (2 oz) slice	140	26.5
Cheesecake, 75 g (3 oz) slice	300	30.0
Chocolate, 25 g (1 oz), milk or plain	150	30.0
Chips, average, 100 g (3½ oz)	250	15.0
Chips, oven, 100 g (3½ oz)	180	10.0
Crisps, 1 x 25 g (1 oz) pack	135	37.0
Crisps, lower fat, 1 x 25 g (1 oz) packet	110	26.0
Croissant, 1 small	165	20.0
Doughnut, 1 jam	225	16.0
Eclair, 1 chocolate	150	24.0
Fruit pie, 125 g (4½ oz) portion	350	10.0
Ice cream, vanilla, 50 g (2 oz) portion	100	7.0
Jam, 10 ml (2 teaspoons)	20	#
Scone, fruit, 1	160	15.0
Sugar, 5 ml (1 teaspoon)	20	#
Sweets, boiled, per 100 g (3½ oz)	327	#
Toffees, per 100 g (3½ oz)	400	17.0

——ALCOHOL——

Alcohol contains no fat, but is high in calories because it contains a type of simple carbohydrate.

	Calories	Per cent of fat content by weight
Beer, 275 ml (10 fl oz, 1/2 pint)	90	#
Lager, 275 ml (10 fl oz, 1/2 pint)	90	#
Spirits, all, 1 measure	50	#
Stout, 300 ml (11 fl oz) can	100	#
Wine, white, medium, 140 ml (5 fl oz, 1/4 pint)	100	#
Wine, white, dry, 140 ml (5 fl oz, 1/4 pint)	90	#
Wine, white, sweet, 140 ml (5 fl oz, 1/4 pint)	140	#
Wine, red, 140 ml (5 fl oz, 1/4 pint)	100	#